D. Baykut, A. Krian (Eds.) ■ **Current Perspectives of the Extracorporeal Circulation**

D. Baykut · A. Krian
Editors

Current Perspectives of the Extracorporeal Circulation

Foreword by K. H. Leitz

STEINKOPFF
DARMSTADT

Springer

Editors' addresses:
Dr. D. Baykut
Prof. Dr. A. Krian
Clinic of Thoracic and Cardiovascular Surgery
Heart Center Duisburg
Gerrickstr. 21
D-47137 Duisburg
Germany

Die Deutsche Bibliothek - CIP-Einheitsaufnahme
Current perspectives of the extracorporeal circulation / D. Baykut; Arno Krian (eds.). With a forw. by K.-H. Leitz. - Darmstadt: Steinkopff; New York: Springer, 2000
ISBN 978-3-7985-1214-6 ISBN 978-3-642-57721-5 (eBook)
DOI 10.1007/978-3-642-57721-5

Medical Editor: Beate Rühlemann - English Editor: Mary K. Gossen
Production: Heinz J. Schäfer
Cover design: Erich Kirchner, Heidelberg
Typesetting: K+V Fotosatz, Beerfelden

Printed on acid-free paper

Preface

The rapid technical improvement of the extracorporeal circulation in the past decades has led to safer, more comfortable and more compatible operations in cardiac surgery and interventions which used to be an adventure are now routine practice. Although most technical variables can easily be accommodated today, the physical influence of artificial circulation systems on blood and tissue still remains uncertain in many cases.

One of our main observations in the use of the extracorporeal circulation is that the prolonged interaction with unphysiological surfaces and forces often releases a cascade of blood and tissue reactions, resulting in a complex type of "disease". Thus, the symptoms can range from unspecific pulmonary inflammations to a severe renal failure or from coagulation problems to a heavy cerebrovascular stroke.

Based on these facts, an interdisciplinary workshop named "Current Perspectives of the Extracorporeal Circulation" took place in Duisburg, Germany on March 26, 1999.

The rationale behind the word "interdisciplinary" was to make a step forward to establish a joint field of knowledge which would be capable of linking the experiences and transfer the know-how of various specialists like cardiac surgeons, neurologists, physiologists or the healthcare industry with their contributions to this essential topic from different perspectives.

In keeping with the concept of the workshop, this book presents the studies of the authors in three main chapters. Chapter 1 reveals the effects of blood-material interaction. Hematological and tissue-related reactions induced by the extracorporeal circulation are discussed in Chapter 2. Finally, Chapter 3 deals with significant clinical aspects.

We hope that this book will makes a wide spectrum of information about the extracorporeal circulation available and accessible. The editors are deeply grateful to all of the authors who contributed to the remarkable success of the meeting. Our special thanks go to Dr. P. Tossios and Mr. S. Hennes for their tireless help in the organization and management of the workshop and to Mr. B. Oedekoven for his valuable editorial support.

Duisburg, November 1999

D. Baykut, M.D.
A. Krian, M.D.

Foreword

Every day thousands of operations are carried out with the heart-lung machine. It is assumed and taken for granted that they will be successful. Very few people are aware of the true complexity of these operations which require an absolute team approach from surgeons, anaesthetists and cardiotechnicians. Each of these three professional groups is responsible for complex processes, in particular when dealing with extracorporeal circulation.

Initially, the heart-lung machine was regarded as being an aid in maintaining the oxygenation, in eliminating carbon dioxide as well as in haemodynamics. We have learned in the last few years that completely different processes also take place. For example, the contact system, the intrinsic and extrinsic coagulation system, the fibrinolytic system and the complement system are activated. The large number of activated mediators have reverse effects on the thrombocytes, endothel cells, neutrophiles monocytes and lymphocytes, i.e. the extent of the biological reaction is considerably greater than was originally assumed. In addition the activated cells can be embolized in various organ systems so that the clinical picture is extremely colourful. The word has been of post-perfusion syndrome or from systemic inflammation reaction syndrome (SIRS). Everyone is also aware of the neurological and neurophysiological dysfunctions after heart operations or the disturbances of the kidney and pulmonary functions or the gastrointestinal tract which, in the worst case, may lead to multiple organ failure after operations. These factors remain extremely serious, but thankfully very rare, complications after open heart operations.

It is thanks to the Duisburg work group that experts from clinics and academia from throughout Europe have been brought together to discuss the aforementioned topic. In addition to the exact analysis of the phenomena which may occur during extracorporeal circulation, talks focus on improvements in everyday practice, e.g. the avoidance of blood-air contact through minimisation of suction or through the use of closed systems. The future will show whether the off-pump movement is the answer to all these questions. As a large number of questions remain open, this symposium should be repeated and the congress publication which has been presented here should be widely distributed to encourage research.

Bremen, November 1999 K.H. Leitz, M.D.

Contents

III. Clinical aspects

Rheological effects of blood-material interactions in extracorporeal circulation

K. Mottaghy
Department of Physiology, University Hospital Aachen, Germany

Introduction

Extracorporeal circulation (ECC) consists of a large variety of applied biomaterials with different geometries and, therefore, with their own flow characteristics. For example, an oxygenator applied in cardiac surgery with the same design shows a different flow characteristic than the same device applied for extracorporeal lung support. On the other hand, ECC is used for different therapeutic applications and hence the artificial device could be quite different: hemodialyzers, heart assist devices, or hybrid organs for liver support. Common components might be tubes, filters, connectors, and reservoirs. Since the demands on the devices are different, different biomaterials must be applied and these have to meet different mechanical strains. Therefore, a large number of different materials are applied: PVC, polyurethane, polycarbonate, polypropylene, silicone etc. There is a consensus about the definition of blood compatibility, which is related to blood material or blood-device interactions (8): "This is the ability of a material, device or system to perform without a clinically significant host response in a specific application". This ability is, however, in tight connection to the fluid dynamic characteristics of flowing blood. The growth rate of thrombi, hemolysis, platelet and leukocyte activation, adsorption of proteins, and more are affected by blood flow conditions.

One should remember that even in the natural body the blood flow characteristics (6, 19) are already considered. Mechanical properties and endothelial activities are different in arterial and venous vessels. High shear stresses, recirculation regions, and prolonged residence times of blood with biomaterials are among other important facts which should be avoided during extracorporeal circulation (20). The aim of this contribution is to consider some rheological aspects which affect the interaction with biomaterials in extracorporeal circulation using basic fluid dynamic models.

Flow models

The components and artificial devices in ECC possess complicated geometrical shapes from the point of view of the determination of precise rheological characteristics. However, the use of some basic fluid dynamic models is useful in order to approach or estimate the hemorheological effects.

Shear flow

We consider a fluid with dynamic viscosity η contained between two large parallel plates of area A, which are separated by a very small distance h. By moving the upper plate with force F and velocity v, the fluid is sheared and has a linear velocity profile as shown in Fig. 1 A. The relation between shear stress τ (=F/A) and shear rate G (velocity gradient) and the dynamic viscosity of the fluid is known as Newton's law of friction (viscosity):

$$\tau = \eta \cdot G \tag{1}$$

Generally, fluids which obey such a relationship are known as Newtonian fluids, e.g., water. Fluids that do not obey this simple relationship are known as non-Newtonian fluids (primarily pastes, slurries, and high molecular weight polymers). Blood also exhibits a non-Newtonian behavior (see below).

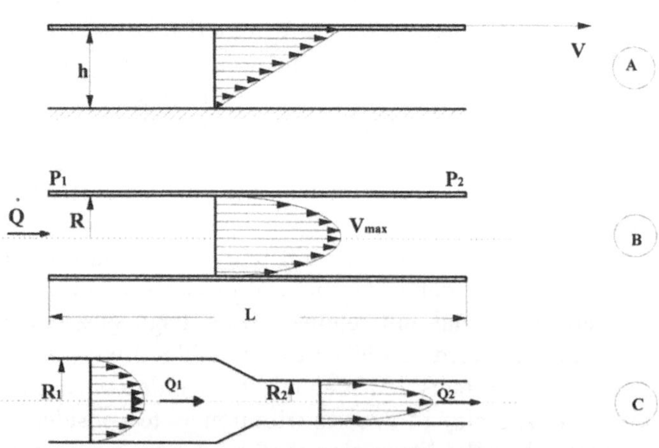

Fig. 1. Schematic drawing of flow models. (A) shear flow, (B, C) pipe flow.

Cylindrical tubes

A lot of ECC components, e.g., tubes have a cylindrical geometry with different diameters (Fig. 1 B und C).

The flow properties for a fully developed laminar flow in a circular tube is known as Poiseuille flow (9):

$$\dot{Q} = \frac{\pi \cdot \Delta p \cdot R^4}{8 \cdot L \cdot \eta} \tag{2}$$

$\dot{Q}$ is flow rate, Δp pressure gradient (p_1–p_2), R radius, L length, and η viscosity of the fluid. The mean velocity (v_m) of the fluid can be calculated from the flow rate and the cross sectional area (A) of the tube.

$$\dot{Q} = A \cdot v_m \tag{3}$$

In case of extension or narrowing of a tube, the established mean velocities can be calculated by means of a continuity relationship (since flow rate remains constant).

$$\dot{Q} = A_1 \cdot v_{m1} = A_2 \cdot v_{m2} \tag{4}$$

Shear rate and shear stress can be calculated as follows:

$$G = \frac{4 \cdot v_m}{R} \tag{5}$$

$$\tau = \frac{4 v_m \cdot \eta}{R}. \tag{6}$$

Channel flow

Channel flow is another example of a typical flow model for some ECC elements. It is a flow between two parallel plates separated with a distance h. This flow model may be applied for rectangular cross sections, e.g., the space between the plates as membranes or heat exchangers. Shear rate and shear stress are described by the following equations:

$$G = \frac{3 v_m}{2h} \tag{7}$$

$$\tau = \frac{3 v_m \cdot \eta}{2h}. \tag{8}$$

Viscosity of blood

As previously mentioned, blood as a fluid shows non-Newtonian behavior. The viscosity of such non-Newtonian fluids is described as the "apparent viscosity" for any given shear condition. Blood is an emulsion (rather than a suspension) of deformable corpuscular cells. Red blood cells (erythrocytes) have at rest a biconcave shape with a diameter of 7.5 μm and a thickness of 2.5 μm. The deformability of erythrocytes enables them to pass through the microcirculation capillaries with a diameter less than 7 μm by means of a "parachute" shape change. This capability of deformation of erythrocytes allows them to have an "active participation" in blood flow. The viscosity of whole blood is flow dependent, which means it is not a constant value in contrast to water or plasma. In larger vessels or tubes in regions of very low flow rates (stasis), the erythrocytes aggregate and form the so-called rouleauxs. The viscosity of blood becomes very high (theoretically infinite) in such regions. At higher shear rates, the cells disaggregate and, because of their deformability and adaptation to the flow, the blood viscosity is reduced considerably. This behavior at physiological ranges is very useful since less energy is required to pump the blood at high flow rates or, in other words, they overcome the flow resistances more easily. In addition, this leads to an increase of gas exchange (11). However, very high shear stresses lead to sublethal or direct cell damage and, in the case of erythrocytes, to hemolysis (3, 4). Figure 2 shows schematically the relationship between blood viscosity and shear forces mentioned previously. It should be noted that the viscosity

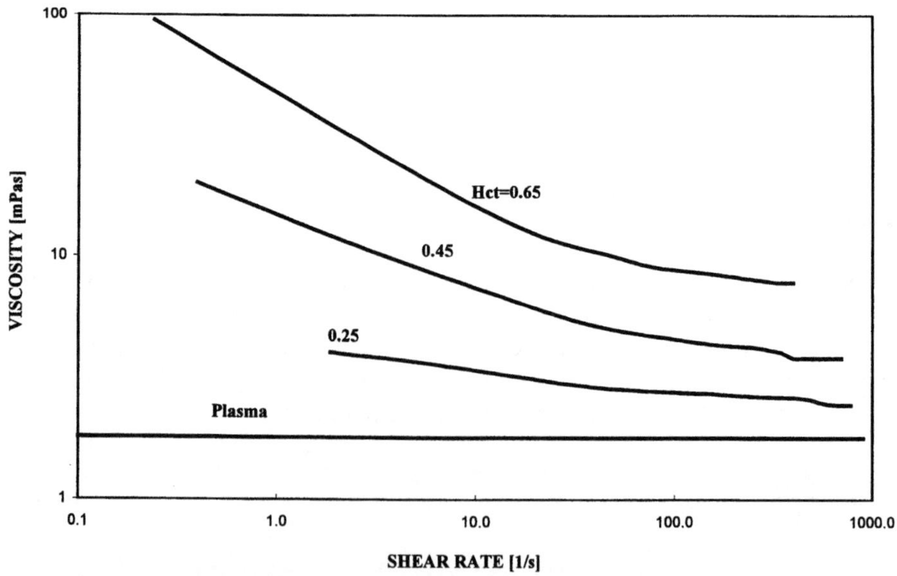

Fig. 2. Relationship between blood viscosity and shear rate; the viscosity of plasma is assumed as 1.8 mPas. Modified in accordance to (11, 18)

of whole blood is also a function of the hematocrit value. At any given shear rate, viscosity is increased by raising hematocrit values. It is evident that for a more precise calculation of the shear stresses occurring in extracorporeal components, the viscosity of blood should not be considered a constant value in Equation 1, but should be measured for any individually used blood and any given flow rate and geometry which determine the shear rate. For practical purposes, however, the data in the literature can be used (5, 11, 18). Figure 3 demonstrates the differences in calculated shear stresses as a function of blood flow rate in the tubes with different inner diameters, calculated using Equations 5 and 6. It is shown that at low blood flow rates there is no linear relationship between obtained shear stress and blood flow rate if the actual blood viscosity is used. Furthermore, the shear stress values are always higher than those calculated using a constant value for plasma viscosity. Table 1 shows an example for natural vessels. Many authors, however, approach the problem by using plasma viscosity for all shear rates. The val-

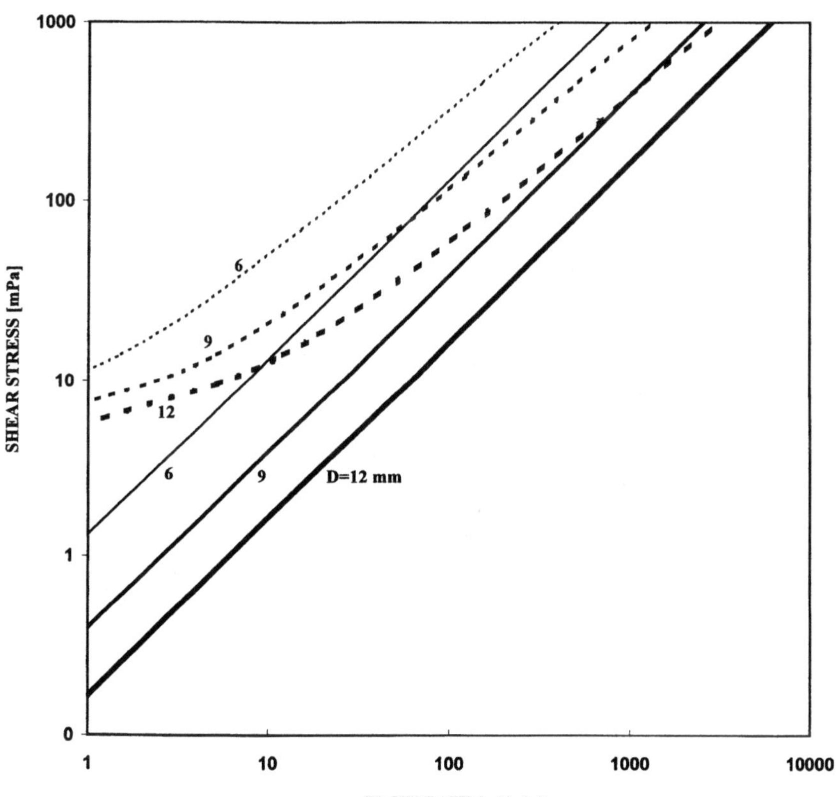

Fig. 3. Relationship between shear stress and blood flow rate through three tubes with different inner diameters. Solid lines: Blood viscosity is presented by a constant value and is assumed to be 1.8 mPas; dashed lines show the same course with actual blood viscosity obtained at the according shear rates as shown in Fig. 2.

Table 1. Typical values of venous flow parameters of dog. Data from (7)

VESSEL	Diameter [cm]	Velocity [cm/s]	Wall shear rate [1/s]
Venules	0.003	0.07	190
Small veins	0.015	1.3	700
Large veins	0.6	3.6	50
Venae cavae	1.25	33.0	210

ues used for plasma viscosity in the literature vary between 1.2 to 3 mPas. Values of up to 5 mPas have also been used in order to approximate the whole blood viscosity. The viscosity of blood has been largely investigated in recent decades. A wide range of parameters affect the blood viscosity (5, 18). An important phenomenon is the axial migration of deformed erythrocytes (Fåhraeus-Lindqvist effect). It becomes evident in capillaries with less than 300 μm diameter. In a plasma layer, the erythrocytes move in the direction of the capillary axis and reduce the effective viscosity of blood. This effect and the influence of temperature changes during extracorporeal circulation with capillary membrane oxygenators (CMO) might play an important role in design and abolishing involved problems.

Contact phase

The surface-induced activation of the blood (contact activation) is a major problem of EC systems. The contact phase is introduced by initial contact period and afterwards the blood is recirculated through the components of ECC up to the finishing of therapy or organ assistance. The components possess different prime volumes and surface areas resulting in different flow velocities and contact time periods with the biomaterial. This is a very important fact for evaluation of hemocompatibility also for in vitro investigations. Figure 4 shows a typical example for the relationships between prime volume V, surface area A, and the duration of first contact (initial) time with blood. Schematic examples are given for a short piece of tube (e.g., connector), a catheter inside a natural vessel (contacting blood from both sides), and a single capillary from a capillary membrane oxygenator. In these configurations the initial contact time varies from 0.04 to 3 s, blood volume from 0.009 to 3 ml, and the total surface area from 1.3 to 12.6 cm^2. It is worthy to note that the piece of the connector has equal surface area as the catheter but equal flow rate to the CMO. In Table 2, estimated values for different components are compiled. For the extracorporeal CO_2 removal method (ECO_2-R), two CMOs are considered resulting in higher surface areas and lower blood flow rates. The contact index (contact time/surface area) is introduced as a parameter which might be useful by comparing biomaterial conduits with different prime volumes and surface areas.

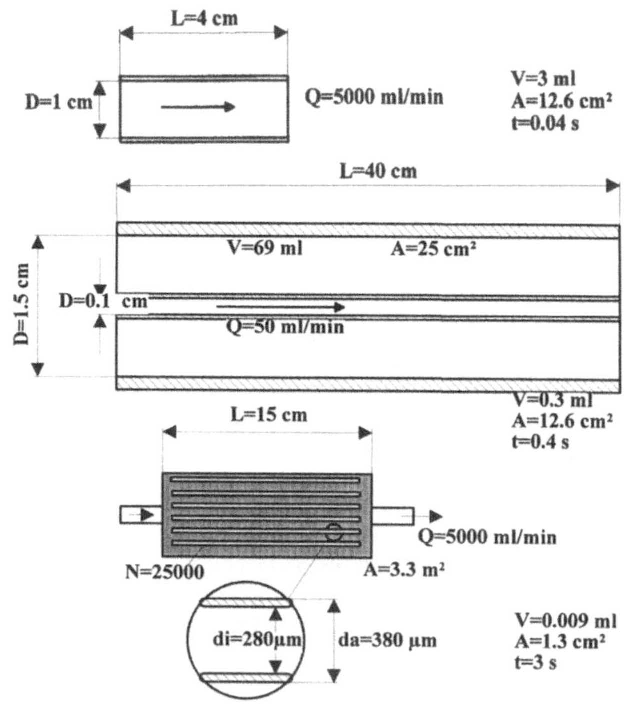

Fig. 4. Examples for the relationship between prime volume (V), total surface area, and initial contact time (t) for a piece of tube (top), an inserted blood catheter (middle), and a single capillary of N-capillaries of a CMO (blood flows inside).

Table 2. Comparison of some relevant parameters in ECC (see text). In the case of extracorporeal CO_2-removal, it is assumed that two identical CMOs are used and the flow rate is as usual in cardiac surgery

	Blood flow rate [l/min]	Surface area [m^2]	Prime volume [ml]	Shear rate [1/s]	Initial contact time [s]	Index time/area [s/m^2]
Oxygenators						
Cardiac surgery	5.0	2.0	400	2000	3	1.5
ECO_2-R	2.0	4.0	800	400	12.5	3.12
Dialyzer	0.2	1.5	115	400	23.6	15.7
Tubing						
Cardiac surgery	5.0	0.03	71	988	0.9	30
ECO_2-R	2.0	0.03	71	395	2.1	70
Dialysis	0.2	0.02	32	130	9.6	480
Housing filters…						
Cardiac surgery	5.0	0.4	1500			
ECO_2-R	2.0	0.4	500			
Dialysis	0.2	0.1	100			

Turbulence and secondary flows

The above mentioned relationship of Poissouille flow is valid for an "ideal" fluid with a laminar flow and a minimum of resistance. The resistance is increased if the flow becomes turbulent. The Reynolds number (Re) describes the ratio of the inertia force to the viscous force in the flow.

$$\mathrm{Re} = \frac{2R \cdot v_m \cdot \rho}{\eta} \tag{9}$$

ρ is the density of the fluid.

In a generalized form, it can be given for a tube flow as follows:

$$\mathrm{Re} = \frac{8 \cdot \rho \cdot v_m^2}{\tau_w} \tag{10}$$

The Re number is dimensionless, and by exceeding a "turnover" point a turbulent flow can be established. The value of this point depends on smoothness of the material and the viscosity of the fluid. A laminar flow in pipes is suggested (23) as become turbulent for Re >2320. In the tubes of ECC together with integrated connectors with their extension or bifurcates, in the arterial blood filter, oxygenator inlet and other parts, the local disturbance at these regions the resistance is raised. Extension and bifurcation of tubes and stenosis perpendicularly changed flow directions lead to recirculations, "dead water" zones, and stagnation flows. A less optimally designed arterial blood filter is a good example for the production of all these flow formations. These kinds of flow possibilities in addition to the main flow stream are depicted schematically in Fig. 5. Detailed reports about the fluid dynamics of such kinds of flow properties can be found in (10).

Blood-material interaction

It is evident that the blood-material interaction is not simply effected by overall blood flow, surface structure, and chemical properties of the biomaterial, but it is important to pay attention to local details in the material walls.

Another important effect is the necessity of using an antithrombotic agent, usually heparin, in association with polymers in extracorporeal circuits. Therefore, the consideration of the anticoagulation effect itself (1, 12, 25) is very important in connection with the interrelationship between blood flow and biomaterial. A general overview of this interrelationship is shown in Fig. 6: the anticoagulated blood flows with a flow rate in the range of cardiac output or less first through catheters and tubes and is pumped through the artificial devices. Depending on the application of ECC, the passage of blood through filters, reservoirs, etc. is necessary. After this first contact with all of

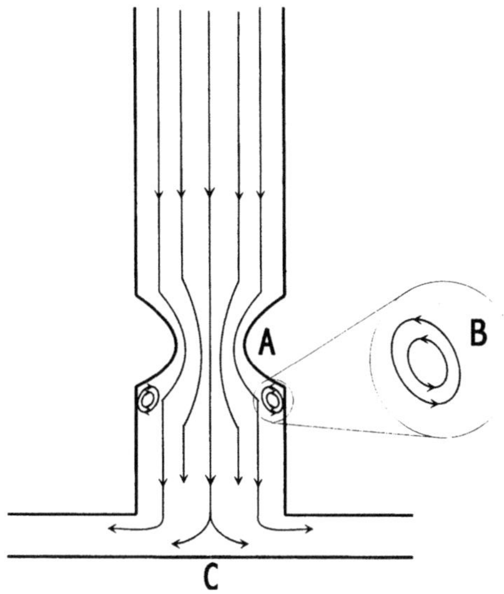

Fig. 5. Schematic presentation of stenosis (A), secondary flow (B), bifurcation and stagnation (C) in accordance with (10, 19).

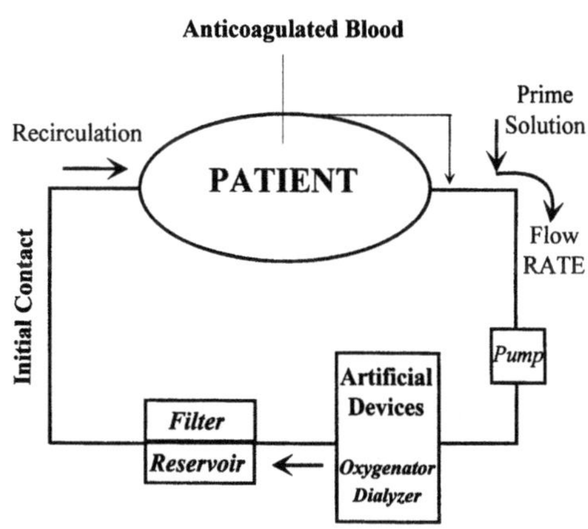

Fig. 6. Schematic drawing demonstrating the interaction of blood flow and biomaterial contact.

the surfaces, the blood is recirculated again through the ECC. The geometry of the artificial device and the other components determine the local flow situation, the contained blood volume, and the contact duration. The local flow situation is characterized by different blood flow velocities, and different wall shear stress values, laminar or turbulent flow, and generation of secondary flows in addition to main flow direction. The consideration of wall shear stress is important for the degree and alteration of plasma protein adhesion and cell alterations. In the main flow stream, the shearing of blood and secondary flows are the processes which effect (besides the cell alterations) the degree of aggregation (especially of thrombocytes), the collision rate, and the diffusion rate of other components, especially blood coagulation factors and anticoagulants. It is evident that these disturbances may not interact with their biomaterials surface in the same place. Moreover, they are carried by flow and interact with the surface in other parts of the ECC components by recirculation in the body and again to the extracorporeal system.

Assessment of biocompatibility

For evaluation of hemocompatibility of artificial devices and the integrated components, in vitro and animal testing are the usual procedures. Because of the therapeutic interventions and lack of standardization during clinical studies the interpretation of results is difficult. Animal experiments can be designed to obtain more defined boundary conditions. But differences in blood properties, e.g., thrombocyte activity (24), of animals do not allow an exact comparison to human blood. In vitro studies allow investigations with human blood. Since the amount of donated blood is limited, an in vitro study with complete components of the ECC system with a single donor is not feasible. Therefore, the design of a reasonable in vitro circuit and the choice of ECC components is still the subject of investigation (14). Examples are recirculation of ECC tubes by means of pumps or pumpless (Chandler loop) systems to study the biocompatibility of different tube polymers (7, 17). Pump-driven circuits can be extended, e.g., by application of a single oxygenator. More local effects can be isolated and investigated by application of shear flow "viscometers". Shear flows are often used in order to investigate the effect of shear stress by changing the shear rate. This kind of shear flow (see Fig. 1 A) can be realized by means of two concentric cylinders or by a cone-plate viscometer.

Blood flowing through artificial organs or stenosis can be subjected to high shear forces for very short times. The effect of high shear forces up to 255 N/m^2 for exposure times shorter than 700 ms are reported (26) in order to investigate the red blood cells and platelets, and trauma alterations.

The most interesting publications reported in recent years deal with the effect of defined fluid dynamic shear upon platelet aggregates and neutrophil adhesion (21, 22). As expected shear stress dependencies are found in certain ranges of shear stresses. But it is also shown how complex the subject becomes when one takes into consideration the effect of receptor biology, e.g., adhesion receptors, fibrinogen cross-bridging receptors, ADP, etc. The results demonstrate how difficult it is to approach the problem theoretically and design hydrodynamic models to prove it. It should be mentioned that these kinds of investigations are usually carried out with, for example, platelet-rich plasma or other cell suspensions in order to standardize the boundary conditions. Furthermore, the direct effect of the biomaterial is neglected here. A new approach for a shear dependence of whole blood with disposable blood-contacting materials may deliver more information about the interaction of sheared blood and the biomaterial (14). Another interesting theoretical consideration on coagulation on biomaterials in flowing blood is reported in (2). This is one of the more rare publications which studies the role of blood flow on the transport of coagulation factors to the biomaterial surface or away from them. It is emphasized that the contact phase compromises about 50 reactions which occur during the first 100–200 s of initial contact, and because of physical and biochemical complexity, the ideal non-thrombogenic material might be impossible to find. This statement is in accordance with the increased interest of surface modification in the last ten years. It should be remembered that natural blood vessels are active surfaces. Here are natural agents produced or released, e.g., antithrombin III, prostacycline, heparin, etc., which "work" against the possible disturbances of blood substitutes or blood flow behavior and modulate the natural contact phase activation. The introduction of covalently bounded heparin to the biomaterials (16) was probably a milestone in this direction. This is the first step to generate an endothelium-like material. Experimental and clinical investigations have proved the efficacy of this idea (12, 16).

Concluding remarks

Hemocompatibility of the biomaterials of ECC components is largely dependent upon the fluid dynamic properties of the devices. For further improvements, the local flow properties should be taken into consideration. However, the precise understanding of the coagulatory problems that occur in the extracorporeal circuits is limited by our present knowledge of the cellular, molecular, and physiological mechanisms. There is still a great need for more relevant flow models and measuring parameters.

Present work on tissue-engineering research may deliver new "hybrid" surfaces which may compensate for the effects of unpredictable blood flow conditions. However, a more "generalized" surface modification of biomaterials, e.g., with heparin in combination with other anticoagulatory and antithrombogenetic agents in order to mimic a endothelia-like surface may represent a more promising solution for the near future.

References

1. Ansell J, Slepchuk N, Kumar R, Lopez A, Southard L, Deykin D (1980) Heparin induced thrombocytopenia: A perspective study. Thrombo Haemostas 43:61
2. Basmadjian D, Sefton MV, Baldwin SA (1997) Coagulation on biomaterials in flowing blood: some theoretical considerations. Biomaterials 18:1511–1522
3. Bernstein EF, Blackshear PL, Keller KH (1967) Factors influencing erythrocyte destruction in artificial organs. Am J Surgery 114:126
4. Bernstein EF, Gleason LR (1967) Factors influencing haemolysis with roller pumps. Surgery 61:432
5. Dintenfass L (1985) Blood Viscosity Hyperviscosity & Hyperviscosaemia. MTP Press Limited, Lancaster Boston the Hague Dordrecht
6. Fung YC (1997) Biomechanics, Circulation. Springer, New York Berlin Heidelberg
7. Gardner RL (1974) An examination of the fluid mechanics and thrombus formation time parameters in a Chandler rotating loop system. J Lab Clin Med 84:494
8. Gurland HJ, Davison AM, Bonomini V, Falkenhagen D, Hansel S, Kishimoto T, Lysaght MJ, Moran J, Valek A (1994) Definitions and terminology in biocompatibility. Nephrol Dial Transplant 9(2):4–10

9. Hughes WF, Brighton JA (1967) Fluid Dynamics. McGraw-Hill Book Company, New York St Louis San Francisco Toronto Sydney
10. Karino T, Kwong HHM, Goldsmith HL (1979) Particle flow behaviour in models of branching vessels – I. Vortices in 90° T-junctions. Biorheology 16(3):231
11. Mottaghy K, Haest CW, Cremer J, Derissen W (1984) Oxygen uptake into the sheared flowing blood: Effects of red cell membranes and haematocrit. In: Lübbers DW, Acker H, Leniger-Follert E, Goldstick TK (eds) Oxygen Transport to Tissue V. Plenum Publishing Corp, New York, pp 175–185
12. Mottaghy K, Oedekoven B, Bey R, Schmid-Schönbein H (1985) Extracorporeal anticoagulation using a serine protease inhibitor in hemodialysis in sheep. Trans Am Soc Artif Int Organs 31:534–536
13. Mottaghy K, Oedekoven B, Schaich-Lester D, Pöppel K, Küpper W (1989) Application of surfaces with end-point attached heparin to extracorporeal circulations with membrane lungs. Trans Am Soc Artif Int Organs 35:146–152
14. Mottaghy K, Kirberich S: Effect of sheared blood and secondary flow on foreign surfaces (in preparation)
15. Oedekoven B (2000) Biocompatibility research on extracorporeal components. In: Baykut D (ed) Current Perspectives of the Extracorporeal Circulation. Steinkopff, Darmstadt, pp 13–22
16. Olsson P, Larm O, Larsson R, Lins E, Swedenborg J (1983) Requirements for thromboresistance of surface-heparinized materials. Ann NY Acad Sci 416:525–537
17. Rhodes NP, Kumary TV, Williams DF (1996) Influence of wall shear rate on parameters of blood compatibility of intravascular catheters. Biomaterials 17:1995–2002
18. Schmid-Schönbein H, Wells RE (1971) Rheological properties of human erythrocytes and their influence upon the "anomalous" viscosity of blood. Ergeb Physiologie 63:147–219
19. Schmid-Schönbein H (1988) Thrombose als ein Vorgang in „strömendem Blut". Hämostaseologie 8:149–172
20. Schmid-Schönbein H, Wurzinger LJ (1995) Enzyme Activation in Blood Perfused Artificial Organs. Martinus Nijhoff Publishers, the Hague Boston London
21. Tandon P, Diamond SL (1997) Hydrodynamic effects and receptor interactions of platelets and their aggregates in linear shear flow. Biophysical J 73:2819–2835
22. Taylor AD, Neelamegham S, Hellums JD, Smith CW, Simon SI (1996) Molecular dynamics of the transition from L-selectin- to β_2-integrin-dependent neutrophil adhesion under defined hydrodynamic shear. Biophysical J 71:3488–3500
23. Truckenbrodt E (1968) Strömungsmechanik. Springer, Berlin Heidelberg New York
24. Wurzinger LJ, Baldauf W, Tobias E, Mottaghy K (1979) Species differences in platelet aggregation with special reference to heparin as anticoagulant. In: Schmid-Schönbein H, Teitel P (eds) Basis Aspects of Blood Trauma. Martinus Nijhoff Publishers, the Hague Boston London, pp 80–97
25. Wurzinger LJ, Schmid-Schönbein H (1981) Species differences in platelet aggregation and the influence of citrate and heparin anticoagulation thereon. ASAIO J 4:149–156
26. Wurzinger LJ, Opitz R, Blasberg P, Schmid-Schönbein H (1985) Platelet and coagulation parameters following millisecond exposure to laminar shear stress. Thrombo Haemost 54(2):381–386

Author's address:
Prof. Dr. K. Mottaghy
Institut für Physiologie
Medizinische Fakultät RWTH Aachen
Pauwelsstr. 30
D-52057 Aachen
Germany

Biocompatibility research on extracorporeal components

B. Oedekoven
Department of Physiology, University Hospital Aachen, Germany

Introduction

Apart from functional, technical, and safety aspects, the biocompatibility of extracorporeal circuit components has become a very important demand. Oxygenators, reservoirs, and arterial filters as well as other components like tubing and connectors consist of many different polymers. Each must be chosen regarding functional properties and the suitability for the manufacturing processes. These materials represent of course foreign surfaces for the blood, unavoidably leading to blood reactions with possibly serious systemic consequences. To minimize these unwanted biological effects, polymers are constantly developed and modified in order to meet finally technical and medical demands with the best biocompatibility at the same time. Therefore these biomaterials must become investigated in every respect: (1): technically, e.g., process engineering properties, function, and durability, (2) medically, e.g., the toxicity, side-effects, and last but not least the biocompatibility. The latter is a big challenge due to the large number of polymers and additionally because the original form of biomaterials is usually thermally transformed resulting in individual changes in their biocompatibility properties. Therefore many models must be applied, considering various important factors and conditions resulting from the specific situations of blood/foreign surface contact. Depending on the scientific questions static or dynamic experimental set-ups can be used. Either the basic polymer, e.g., as a flat sheet, or the final product is investigated by measurement of a lot of parameters to characterize the biocompatibility performance.

Devices, components and biomaterials

From the very beginning of heart surgery the use of foreign material was inevitable. At least with regard to their function and purpose, most of the extracorporeally used components are up to now more or less unchanged but the number of the processed materials constantly increased (Table 1). Of course the enormous progress in the fields of process engineering, polymer

Table 1. Examples of components for extracorporeal circuits an the applied biomaterials

Components	Biomaterial
Oxygenators	Polypropylene, silicone, polyurethane
Heat exchangers	Steel, aluminum, polyethylene, polypropylene, polyurethane
Reservoirs	Polyamide, polyester, polysiloxane
Filter	Polyester
Tubing	Polyvinylchloride (PVC), silicone

chemistry, etc., allows nowadays the construction and production of high-tech devices and high-quality disposables for routine clinical applications.

These biomaterials have to meet at first many technical demands to obtain their function and safety. The rather high number results from the very specific purposes for each material as there are, e.g., gas permeability for the oxygenator membranes, rigidity of housings, flexibility of tubing, temperature conductivity of heat exchanger walls or the desired transparency of some components. However, the use of these materials depends not only from their availability and functionality. The economical aspects must not be neglected because all parts of extracorporeal circuits are manufactured as mass products and must fulfill the demands on low cost components. However, there is one additional medical property which makes it much more complicated and expensive: The keyword is "hemocompatibility".

The term "hemocompatibility" was defined as "... the ability of a material, device or system to perform without a clinically significant host response in a specific application" (3). This description of hemocompatibility allows the interpretation of a material property not to be necessarily hemocompatible as an absolute value, but to be relatively better accepted by the blood than others used for the same purpose. That means, hemocompatibility is relative. It depends among further conditions on blood contact time, surface area, volume/surface relation, blood flow, shear rate, and also from the frequency and duration of blood contact to the biomaterial (6).

Demands on in vitro models, test media and parameters

Of course before the clinical application of biomaterials, many expensive investigations are required. This still includes the basic research, the adaptation of analysis methods to specific scientific demands, extensive in vitro testing, and finally animal studies.

As mentioned above the in vitro hemocompatibility testing of biomaterials is one important pre-condition for further applications and for experimental or clinical approval. However, the value of the results achieved by these investigations depends strongly on the applied in vitro models. Exemplary demands on in vitro models that at the first view seem to be rather easy to meet are:

- sufficient blood/surface contact area,
- the exclusion of additional foreign surfaces,
- the use of reasonable blood volumes,
- a reproducibility of the set-up,
- easy handling,
- the measurement of relevant parameters,
- the applicability of original materials,
- the adaptability to specific scientific demands,
- the closeness to clinical application.

Unfortunately some of these demands are mutually exclusive. For example, only a few models offer the opportunity to study exclusively the original material of an oxygenator membrane without any blood contact to further foreign surfaces, or, if clinically relevant conditions as, e.g., blood flow are desired, it is also impossible to apply an easy to handle experimental set-up with a low blood volume. These examples demonstrate that each model is almost a compromise. It offers only limited possibilities to answer scientific questions, and the conditions applied must be standardized and documented in order to assess and to compare the achieved results.

Independent from technical advantages and disadvantages of different in vitro models, the choice of the test fluid is of great importance and influences the results of the question to be answered. Comparative studies, for example, demand very equal starting parameters. In general the use of pooled plasma which is storable for a certain period of time is advantageous. But comparable studies on blood cells, e.g., to investigate shear stress effects require whole blood or cell concentrates, which are limited in storability. Therefore different individuals have to donor their blood, resulting in different starting values and more difficult comparability. Table 2 shows some examples of common test media and some advantages and disadvantages for objectives which have to be recognized for their choice. It can be seen that availability, storability, homogeneity, and anticoagulation are important factors which have to be taken into account for reliable in vitro hemocompatibility investigations.

Another very important pre-condition to characterize the biocompatibility of a biomaterial is the selection of the right measuring parameters. Blood

Table 2. Advantages and limitations to be recognized for the choice of the best test medium for specific in vitro hemocompatibility studies

Plasma	Cells	Whole blood
Specific clotting and/or complement studies	*Shear stress studies*	*Complex cell/plasma/material interaction studies*
Pooling	RBC/PLT's	Heparin or citrate for Anticoagulation
Results more reproducible	Different reagibility	Individual donor reactions
Long-term storable	Short-term storable	Not storable

Table 3. Examples for pathways, parameters, and methods of in vitro hemocompatibility studies

Pathway	Parameter	Method
Clotting system	PTT, TT, ATIII, Fibrinogen, TAT,...	Coagulometer, photometer
Complement system	C3a, C5a, TCC (C5-9 complex)...	ELISA
Blood cells	Cell count, released factors (Hb, PF4, β-TG, elastase...)	Counter, ELISA, flow cytometry

contact to foreign surfaces influences a lot of pathways in the blood including the clotting system, coagulation system, and the blood cells. Many parameters are in vitro measurable and partially referable to clinical situations. Some examples for different pathways, parameters, and applied measuring methods are listed in Table 3.

In vitro models

Non-dynamic models

As already mentioned, each in vitro model represents only a compromise as it cannot meet all exemplary demands at the same time listed above. Therefore the right model has to be chosen from a variety of different possibilities to answer specific questions. For screening investigations and to estimate if a material could be useful as a biomaterial, practical and non-complicated models are applied at first. Typical examples for that are the "Bowry Chamber" or similar chamber systems (1, 2) which allow investigations on flat sheets of polymers (Fig. 1).

The "Bowry Chamber" represents a static test system. The gap between two flat polymer sheets within a Plexiglas chamber, sealed by an o-ring is primed with a small blood volume. In parallel connected chambers allow comparative studies on different materials using blood from a single donor. The use of a rocking platform avoids cell sedimentation. The advantages of this system are the simplicity of application and the requirement of only very small blood volumes.

However, the flat shape of a polymer is usually the exception for components of extracorporeal systems. PVC, polyurethane, polyethylene and others polymers are commonly thermally transformed, e.g., to tubes or hollow fibers. The consequence is changed surface properties resulting in possibly different biocompatibility characteristics. The limitations of the "Bowry Chamber" are that only flat materials can be investigated, further foreign material, e.g., the o-ring, is in contact to the test medium and in addition only blood contact under static conditions, far from practical application can be produced. Nevertheless, it is a useful method which is firmly established for initial biocompatibility investigations.

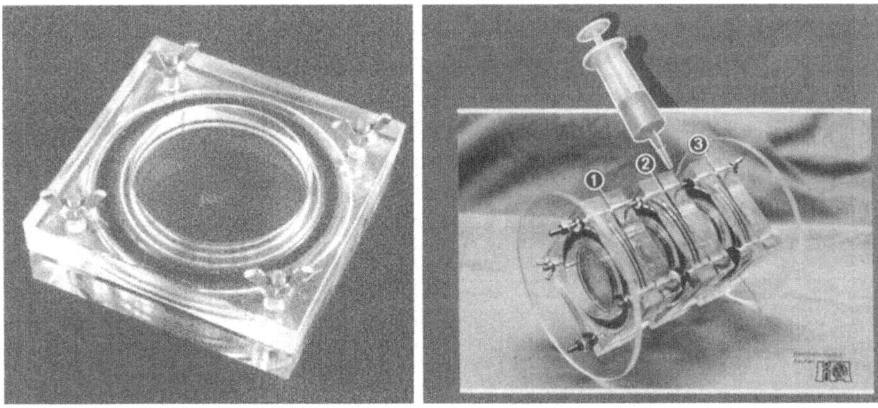

Fig. 1. "Bowry Chamber" modified by Helmholtz-Institut, Aachen, Germany (2). Left: single chamber; right: connected in parallel at a rolling platform to avoid blood cell sedimentation.

In order to investigate tubing for extracorporeal circuits, special in vitro models can be applied. A test system for tubing which is in principle rather similar to the "Bowry Chamber" for polymer sheets is the so-called "rolling platform". Figure 2 shows a schematic drawing of this test system. Pieces of ECC tubing with a certain length are filled with whole blood and clamped at both ends. Blood can be transferred into the tubing directly from the donor, e.g., for special investigations on the function of heparin coatings, or blood is drawn and anticoagulated by citrate or heparin. The tubes are rotated by a "rolling platform" and rotated for a defined period of time until samples are taken for blood investigations. Depending on the objective of the study the tubes can be refilled several times, e.g., to study the heparin leaching kinetics from the coated surfaces or to investigate the effects of protein deposition on blood cells over the time.

In contrast to the "Bowry Chamber" no additional foreign surface is in contact with the blood than the biomaterial to be investigated. Although the investigations on original polymers in their final shape are possible, there is still the disadvantage of having only a static system. Rolling the tubing avoids sedimentation of blood cells but it does not generate flow conditions as in real application. Therefore "Bowry Chamber", "rolling platform" and similar experimental set-ups cannot answer the question how the blood and the biomaterial would react under dynamic conditions. For this purpose other in vitro models must be applied.

Dynamic models

To investigate, for example, surface modified polymers (e.g., heparin coatings), it is of great interest how the surface behaves when exposed to flowing

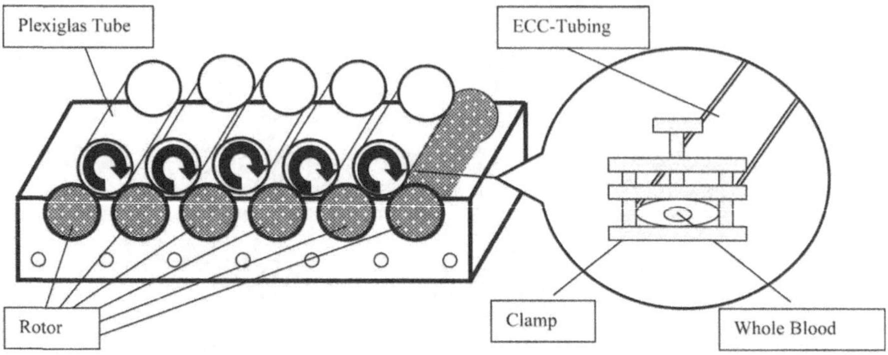

Fig. 2. Left: Schematic drawing of the "rolling platform" with indicated rotating Plexiglas tubes, covering the tubing to be tested. Right: Clamped tubing filled with whole blood as put into Plexiglas tube.

blood. Blood flow in extracorporeal circulation is established by means of pumps with a pulsatile or continuous pump mode. It is obvious that the use of pumps in in vitro models has the advantage of having more realistic conditions. On the other hand, there are also disadvantages which have to be weighed against each other: high shear forces for example generated by roller pumps are a factor which can trigger blood processes and falsify the pure blood/surface interaction. But piston or syringe pumps, avoiding high shear stress peaks, possess foreign surfaces on its own, which may misrepresent the measured effects of the surface to be tested. Figure 3 shows a schematic drawing of roller pumps (a) and a piston pumps application (b) for dynamic investigations of tubing polymers or modules with, e.g., integrated hollow fibers.

The advantage of these pump driven systems are the dynamic blood/surface contact conditions. Disadvantageous is the difficulty to estimate the effects of shear stress and additional foreign surfaces on measured hemocompatibility parameters. Therefore, only plasma, serum or other cell free media can be applied to investigate objectives as complement activation or protein adsorption on foreign surfaces.

Considering these limitations, dynamic hemocompatibility investigations are necessary. In order to study tubing under blood flow conditions without the disturbances of pumps, the "Chandler Loop" system represents a useful alternative to pump driven models. Already in the 50th 1950s Chandler developed this system for basic research on the coagulation system (4). Figure 4a shows schematically a drawing of the "Chandler Loop" principle. A certain volume of blood is filled into tubing which is formed into a closed loop. This loop is mounted to vertically positioned holder and rotates at a defined speed by means of an electric driven motor. Due to gravity the blood remains in the lower part of the loop. The friction at the tubing wall leads to a flow in the direction of the rotating tubing. At each end of the blood column, the blood stream at the walls turns around and becomes a central

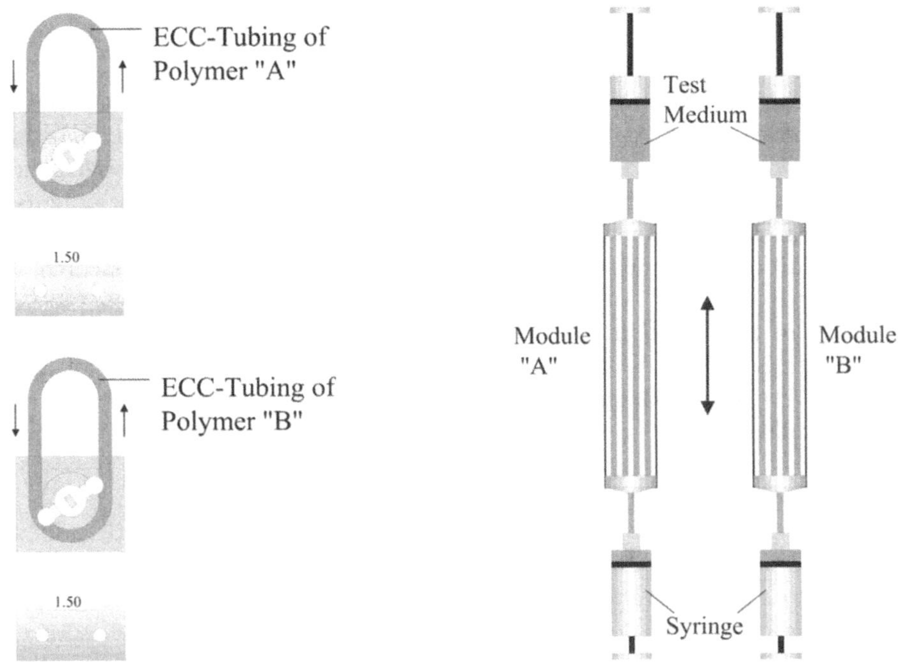

Fig. 3. (a) Set-up with two roller pumps establishing pulsatile flow through ECC tubing to be compared to each other with regard to effects on hemocompatibility, according to (8); (b) Test medium is continuously pushed back and forth through a small scaled dialyzer module with integrated capillary membranes by means of piston or syringe pumps, according to (7).

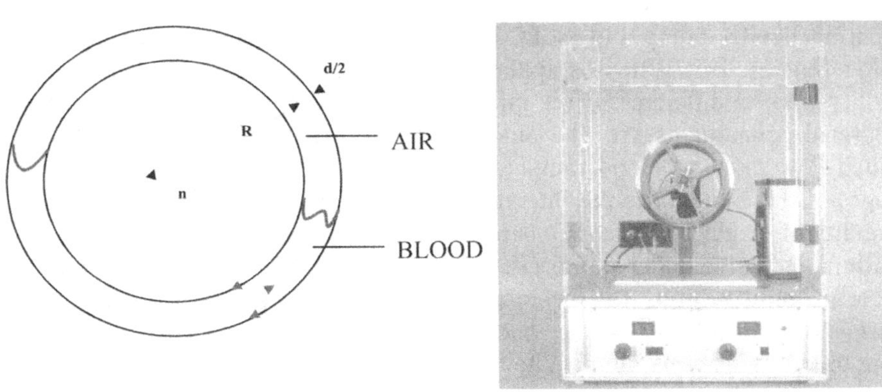

Fig. 4. (a) Left: Principle of the Chandler loop system; (b) Right: Multi-channel Chandler loop device (Dept. of Physiology and IZKF "Biomat", Aachen).

stream in the opposite direction. By this method the blood is brought constantly into contact to the foreign surface without any pump. The laminar flow avoids unwanted shear stress on blood cells.

Figure 4b shows a "Chandler Loop" device, constructed in our department, allowing, e.g., comparative studies on different tubing polymers or surface modifications also with different inner diameters under well standardized conditions. Ten tubings can be investigated simultaneously at adjustable shear rates and temperatures (4).

In addition to comparative hemocompatibility studies, basic research is being performed, e.g., on the kinetics of blood activation processes, the influences of the blood/air interface, and shear stress. As a matter of fact the "Chandler Loop" can be only applied for inner diameter in the range of ECC tubing. Very small diameters, e.g., of vessel catheters, prevent blood flow as, due to adhesion forces, the blood rotates at the same speed as the tubing wall.

In reality, the situation for blood at extracorporeal circulation is much more complicated than it occurs in the in vitro models already described. These models are of advantage for screening new polymers or surface modifications, or for the evaluation of the hemocompatibility of particular components, e.g., with well definable geometry. These investigations are more or less inexpensive and can be, therefore, frequently performed. During this phase of polymer investigations, their development may still change or surface modifications can become optimized.

As a matter of fact, the environment for blood and the conditions with regard to blood flow, shear rates, alternating contact materials, etc. are extremely complex in an extracorporeal system. Here blood is in contact with many different biomaterials; blood flow varies as well as the shear conditions inside oxygenators, filters, reservoirs or tubing. Clinically applied, the sum of the effects from blood/surface contacts and interactions inside all extracorporeal components is of relevance.

In order to simulate those conditions in vitro, a small-scale extracorporeal system can be applied. The so-called "filter loop system" consists of a conventional roller pump and an ECC tubing circuit including an arterial blood filter (Fig. 5). This system is applied to compare the effects on hemocompatibility, e.g., of different surface modifications like heparin coatings for all integrated components (5). The blood is pumped through the system at a defined flow rate and blood samples are taken at regular intervals. The advantages of this system are the integration of all relevant biomaterials, the applicability of original ECC components, the establishment of dynamic flow conditions including roller pump effects and a standardized set-up with reasonable priming volume. On the other hand, this dynamic model is comparatively complicated to handle, and each experimental performance requires the blood unit of one donor. The last is the most important limitation of this in vitro model because no simultaneous tests can be performed as a single donor unit of blood is only enough for priming of one system.

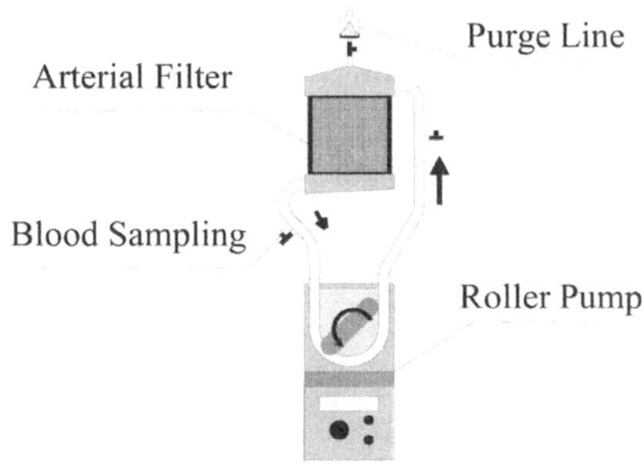

Fig. 5. Schematic drawing of the filter loop system.

Conclusion

A selection of aspects of in vitro hemocompatibility research was briefly reported in order to give an overview on the wide spectrum of objectives, models, and also their limitations. Summarizing it can be concluded that for the assessment of in vitro study results the consideration of many conditions is required to predict probable blood reaction on biomaterials under clinical conditions. It always has to be taken into consideration if static or dynamic blood contact was established, the polymer was tested in its final or in an intermediate shape, which pathways were investigated, the value of the blood flow and wall shear rates contact times and if the results represent an acute response or the kinetics of blood processes (6).

References

1. Cheung AK, Lemke H (1994) Criteria and standardization for biocompatibility. Nephro Dial Transplant 2:72–76
2. Glasmacher-Seiler B, Schnitzler U, Voigt S, Lührs H, Reul H (1993) In vitro blood chamber tests for the investigation of blood-material interactions. Proc VIIth Colloquium on Biomaterials. Aachen
3. Gurland HJ, Davison AM, Bonomini V, Falkenhagen D, Hansen S, Kishimoto T, Lysaght MJ, Moran J, Valek A (1994) Definitions and terminology in biocompatibility. Nephrol Dial Transplant 9:4–10
4. Henseler A, Oedekoven B, Andersson C, Mottaghy K (1999) Entwicklung eines modifizierten "Chandler Loops" zur in vitro Evaluierung der Hämokompatibilität von ECC-Schläuchen. Abstracts 28. Internationale Fortbildungs- und Arbeitstagung der Deutschen Gesellschaft für Kardiotechnik, Würzburg
5. Keldenich S, Kopp R, Kirschfink M, Klein B, Henseler A, Oedekoven B, Mottaghy K (1998) Biocompatibility of different heparin coatings investigated by an new dynamic flow model: A comparative study. ASAIO J 44:3
6. Klinkmann H, Davison AM (1994) The biocompatibility puzzle – partly solved, partly enigmatic. Nephrol Dial Transplant 9:184–186

7. Kushihata S, Yorioka N, Oda H, Ye XF, Yamakido M (1998) Effects of dialysis membranes on the kinetics of tumor necrosis factor-α production by peripheral mononuclear cells in chronic hemodialysis patients. Int J Artif Organs 21/7:383–390
8. Mottaghy K, Oedekoven B, Pöppel K, Kovacs B, Kirschfink M, Bruchmüller K, Kashefi A, Geisen C (1991) Heparin-coated versus non-coated surfaces for extracorporeal circulation. Int J Artif Organs 14/11:721–728

Author's address:
B. Oedekoven
Institut für Physiologie
Medizinische Fakultät
RWTH Aachen
Pauwelsstr. 30
D-52057 Aachen
Germany

Experimental studies in hemo- and biocompatibility of artificial surfaces in cardiovascular surgery

W. Heller and H.P. Wendel
Department of Thoracic and Cardiovascular Surgery,
University of Tübingen, Germany

Introduction

Already in 1890 Brown-Sequard investigated artificial blood circulation to the organs; however decades of basic research were carried out until, in 1954, Gibbon first successfully applied extracorporeal circulation (ECC) to a human with the aid of a heart-lung machine (HLM). In the early days of the development of ECC technology there were questions regarding the efficiency of the individual parts: most importantly the pumps and oxygenators. The plate or grid oxygenators then in use were replaced by the so-called bubble oxygenator. Since the latter functions on a completely different principle of oxygenation, it was not surprising that most of the investigations were conducted on the efficiency of the oxygenation involved. However, very soon both systems displayed problems regards hemolysis which in the end were met through the introduction of membrane oxygenators. When these oxygenators came into use it was not completely clear that they would bring with them a whole new range of problems, namely those of surface contact between the artificial membrane and the blood. Here, at the latest, it was to be shown that the problem of blood clotting and that of contact with artificial surfaces combined to form one big problem area. In recent years, it was thought that a way out of these difficulties had been found through the method of coating the membrane oxygenators with heparin, thus, solving both the problem caused by high heparin dosages and that of surface contact with the blood.

Despite constant improvements in technology and in the medication available, the HLM is still only an insufficient substitute for the physiological circulation (5, 9, 10, 14, 15). A series of pathophysiological occurrences are to be found as a result:

- Hypotension and continued compensated state of shock with disturbances of the macro- and microcirculation at pressures of 60–80 mmHg, registered through kinins which lower the peripheral vascular resistance.
- Reduction of platelet functional activity and partially destruction; leucopenia and hemolysis. These could be caused mainly by mechanical irritation such as turbulence but also through stasis of the blood in the tubing of the HLM. Furthermore, the blood cells are traumatized by the pump, filters, and through suction as well as by the artificial surfaces of the system.

- Contact activation of plasmatic clotting factors and denaturation of proteins through the nonphysiological surfaces of the devices (metal, glass, plastic) instead of the bioinert intima (4).

The central problem with ECC, however, is the activation of the clotting and inflammatory cascade and other plasmatic defense systems particularly responsible for kinin production. Therefore, once the intrinsic system of blood clotting is set in action, the kallikrein formed from prekallikrein reinforces the activity of the clotting system. It also starts up the fibrinolytic and complement systems as well as the release of bradykinin from HMW kininogen which is peripherally vasodilatory and increases permeability, thus, contributing to the above-mentioned drop in blood pressure. This interaction, of course, also activates the plasma-proteinase inhibitors which have a regulatory effect and are responsible for preventing an excessive reaction of the systems (7, 17, 18).

Within the framework of a comparative study, 3 types of pediatric membrane oxygenators of different manufacturers were investigated for their hemocompatibility. The study was carried out simulating clinical conditions using human blood and enlisted the aid of a HLM model developed by us. Thus, an ex vivo model was applied here in order to study the behavior of the parameters of the contact phase and coagulation systems for the stipulated period of 90 minutes of recirculation. This model is also suitable for the study of possible interaction of pharmaceutics indispensible in ECC: heparin and protamine with the cellular compartments of the blood, on the one hand, and the artificial surfaces, on the other. We came to the conclusion that the term "standard heparin" can no longer be maintained. The so-called standard heparins differ to the same extent or more or less from one another as do the low molecular weight heparins (12). For this reason we always used the same optimal high molecular weight heparin in this comparative study.

Materials and methods

In our model (Fig. 1), three types of membrane oxygenators for infants from different companies were compared. Eight oxygenators of each series from these companies (A, B, C) were studied.

Experimental conditions

For 90 min, 500 ml volumes of fully recalcified ACD whole blood (not older than 24 hours) were recirculated in a closed circuit system at 28 °C. Hemodilution and gas flow were regulated in a manner identical to surgical CPB. We used 3.0 IU/ml heparin (Liquemin®, Hoffmann-La Roche, Basel, Switzerland)

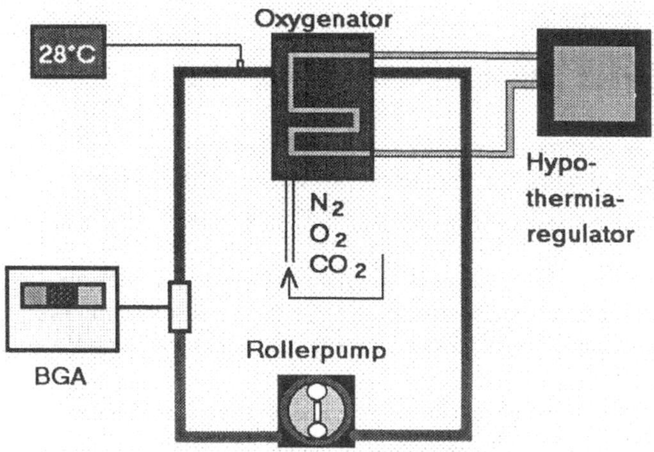

Fig. 1. Example of membrane oxygenator set-up.

in the membrane oxygenators available commercially. The priming volume consisted of 50 ml 5% glucose solution (Delta-Pharma GmbH, Pfullingen, Germany), 116 ml Ringer lactate (Schiwa, Glandorf, Germany), 10 ml $NaHCO_3$, and 24 ml 10% calcium chloride (both from Braun Melsungen AG, Melsungen, Germany). Before priming, the oxygenators and tubing were rinsed in 700 ml Ringer lactate for 30 minutes. A hypothermic regulator maintained the temperature at 28 °C at the arterial exit of the oxygenator. Oxygenation was effected with a mixture of 77% N_2, 20% O_2, and 3% CO_2. Blood samples were taken before circulation and at 1, 5, 10, 30, 60, and 90 minutes after commencement of circulation. After centrifugation, the heparin concentration in each sample was determined and antagonized with protamine chloride (Hoffmann-La Roche, Basel, Switzerland) in a ratio of 1:1 (some contact system assays are influenced by high heparin levels). All plasma samples were shock frozen in liquid nitrogen and stored at -20 °C.

Chromogenic peptide substrate assays for heparin (anti-Xa activity), F XII, kallikrein-like activity, and kallikrein inhibition were performed with kits supplied by Unicorn Diagnostics Ltd. London, UK, or Chromogenix AB Molndal, Sweden. α_1-proteinase inhibitor-PMN elastase complexes (PMN-Elastase-α_1-PI), and platelet factor 4 (PF4) levels were determined using ELISA kits supplied by Merck AG, Darmstadt, Germany and Behring Werke AG, Marburg, Germany, respectively. Hemolysis (free plasma hemoglobin) was determined using a colorimetric assay from Boehringer, Mannheim, Germany. All assays were performed in duplicate according to the manufacturers instructions. All values were corrected for hematocrit. The initial values, which differed according to the individual donors blood were equated to 100% and subsequent samples calculated as a percentage of the initial value. Statistical analysis was performed by the statistics software package SPSS (SPSS Software Inc., Chicago, USA) using the method of univariate analysis of variance.

Results

Contact activation

The comparative study of 3 different types of pediatric oxygenators showed an activation of the factor XII system with the application of Oxy C. This activation of the 1st stage of the contact phase already begins after 1 min of recirculation, that is clinically speaking, at the onset of bypass. The rise is continuous with reference to the 100% initial value and, by the end of 90 minutes recirculation, reaches 20%. With the use, however, of Oxy A or B there is a slight consumption, that is, a drop in factor XII during the period of observation.

On account of these results, it therefore seems of particular interest to take a look at the fragments alpha and beta of the Hagemann factor (Fig. 2). These are measured via their inhibitors, however, as they cannot be registered directly. This represents the only means of tracing the pathway. The behavior of these fragments is identical with both Oxy A and B. Both the values of α-FXIIa and β-FXIIa slightly fall already after one minute recirculation. With the Oxy C, totally different results are gained. At the beginning of recirculation there is a significant rise in the β-FXIIa inhibition. A small decrease occurs toward the end of recirculation. This means that, with the application of Oxy C, the pathway clearly points in the direction of the kallikrein system, that is, indicates strong contact phase activation, whereas with Oxy A and B the pathway more strongly leads to the fibrinolytic system and

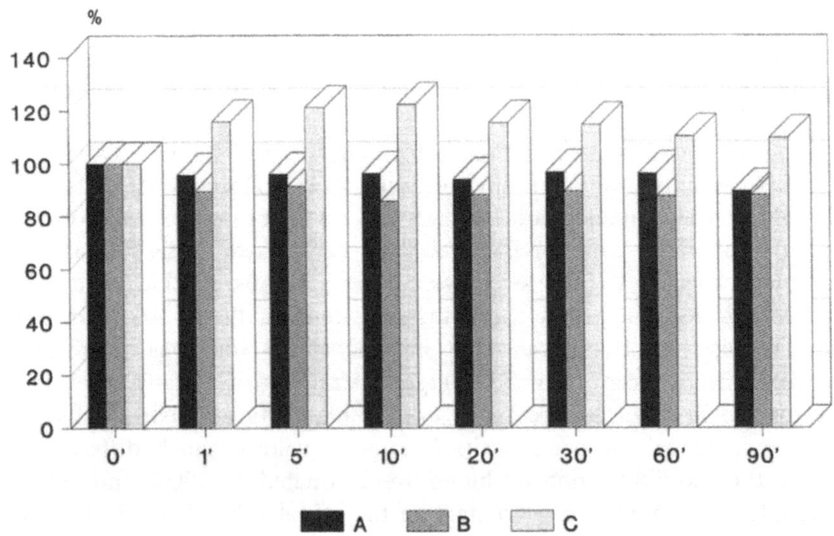

Fig. 2. Beta-factor XIIa-inhibition.

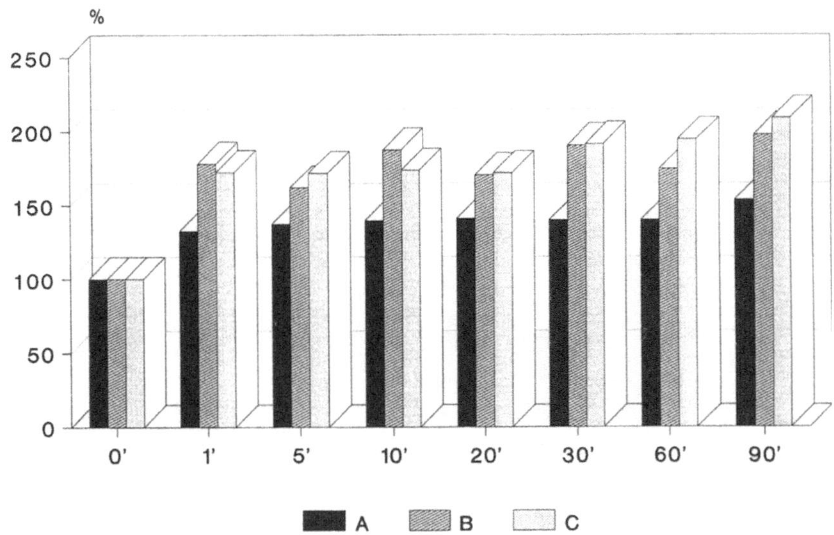

Fig. 3. Kallikrein-like activity.

less to the kallikrein system. This we consider a decisive difference between the sub-groups.

As not otherwise to be expected with the application of Oxy C, there is a significant activation of the kallikrein system already after 1 min recirculation (Fig. 3). This involves a rise from 100% to 200% toward the end of this time (90 min). Unexpected is the equally strong activation that takes place with Oxy B. This result does not correlate with the prekallikrein values. The release of kallikrein (KK) with Oxy A is not significant and is relatively understandable via the PK values. All in all the contact phase activation is at its lowest and not of physiological significance.

Summarising, then, with the application of Oxy C there is a continuous significant activation of the contact phase via the Hageman factor to the KK system.

Cellular components

Hemolysis

Comparing the 3 pediatric oxygenators, the degree of hemolysis (free plasma hemoglobin) as a measure of damage to the erythrocytes gives a different picture from the one described in the contact phase (Fig. 4). The smallest amount of damage to the erythrocytes was registered in the application of Oxy C. After 30 min recirculation, the values for Oxy A and B are already significant and after 60 or 90 minutes, much greater and highly significant (from 100% to 400% or 350%).

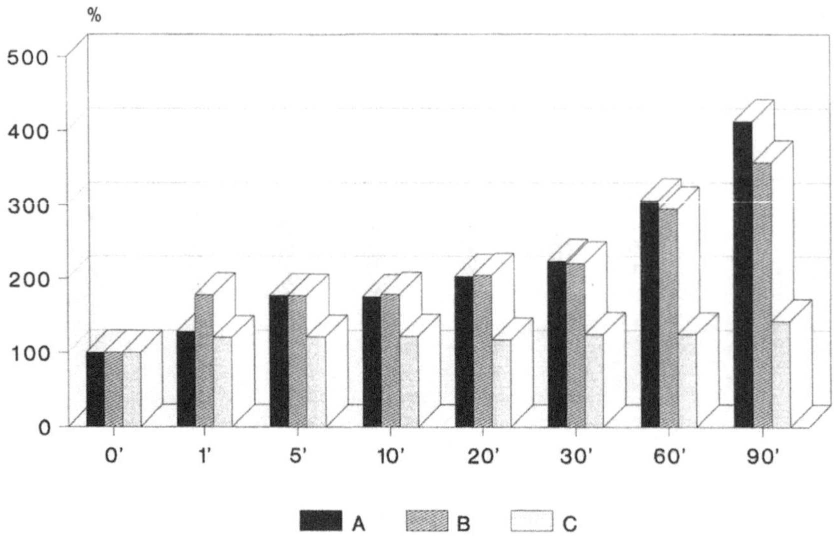

Fig. 4. Hemolysis vs. time.

Platelet factor 4 (PF4)

With the values for this parameter the stronger damaging effect that Oxy A and B have on the cellular components are also reflected (Fig. 5). Thus, already after 1 min of recirculation, the values for these two oxygenators lie significantly higher than the initial values. This is also found to be the case when the values are compared with those for Oxy C. After 90 min of recirculation the values are surprisingly close together for all three oxygenators, i.e., after longer periods of recirculation the 3 oxygenators are roughly the same with regard to their platelet damaging effect.

PMN elastase-α_1-PI

This parameter represents a measure of damage to the neutrophils. Here the differences in the oxygenator runs for Oxy A and B, on the one hand, and Oxy C on the other, can be seen more clearly if the graphical depiction of hemolysis or PF4 is included (Fig. 6). While with Oxy C only a minimal release of PMN elastase is registered, with the application of Oxy A and B already after 10 min of recirculation there is a distinct release of PMN elastase. These values are significantly raised above the initial values after 20 minutes and highly significantly raised after 60 minutes of recirculation. The values for Oxy A after 90 minutes recirculation are lower than those for Oxy B.

All in all, however, there is an extreme difference between Oxy A and B, on the one hand, and Oxy C, on the other, with respect to the granulocyte damage which is represented by the release of PMN elastase.

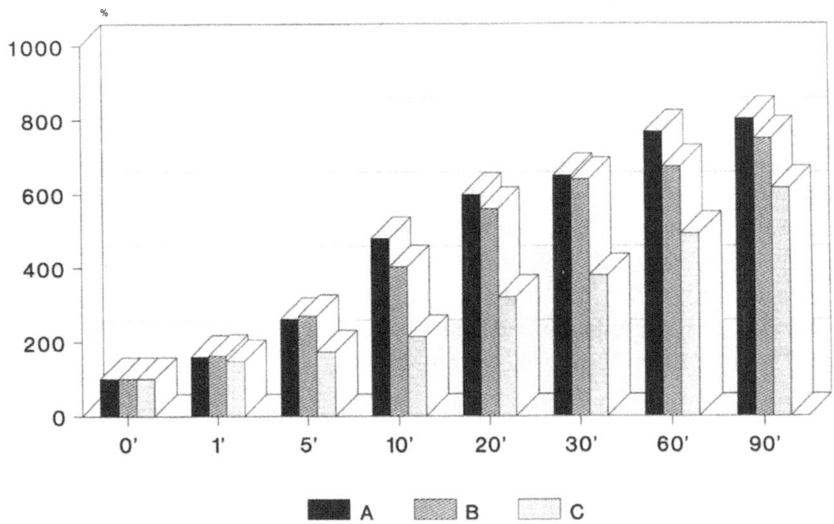

Fig. 5. Platelet factor 4 vs. time.

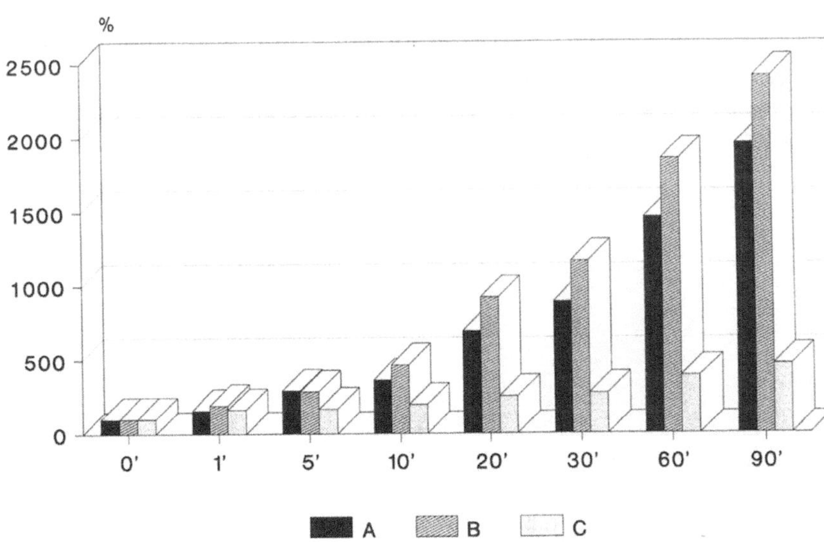

Fig. 6. PMN elastase vs. time.

Coagulation system

TAT

Under the influence of heparin the thrombin that arises forms TAT complexes with AT III (Fig. 7). By measuring the degree of formation of TAT complexes the occurrence of thrombin can be established, as the graphs excellently illustrate. Thus, the behavior of this parameter with Oxy C is especially impressive. After 90 minutes recirculation, the TAT level is highly significant and above the initial value and significantly above the values for Oxy A and B. Significant differences are also to be observed between Oxy A and B after 20 or 30 min of recirculation.

FPA

Since this parameter is also a measure for thrombin generation, FPA is in this way released from fibrinogen through thrombin; thus, it is to be expected that this is the case particularly in the application of Oxy C (Fig. 8). On the whole, this is the case since after 90 min of recirculation the highest FPA was registered which is highly significantly above the initial values. Surprisingly enough similar effects are found with Oxy A. This was not necessarily to be expected due to the TAT levels. All in all then, with Oxy A and C significantly raised FPA values are to be observed in comparison to Oxy B after 60 minutes of recirculation.

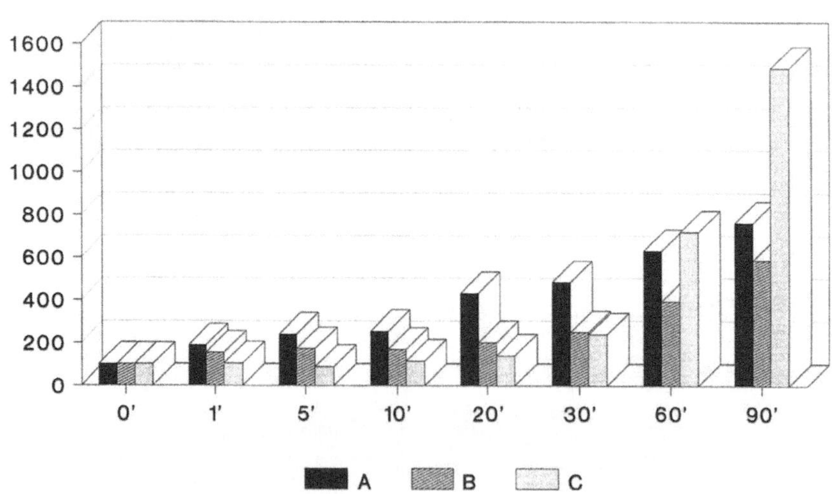

Fig. 7. TAT (thrombin-antithrombin-III-complex) vs. time.

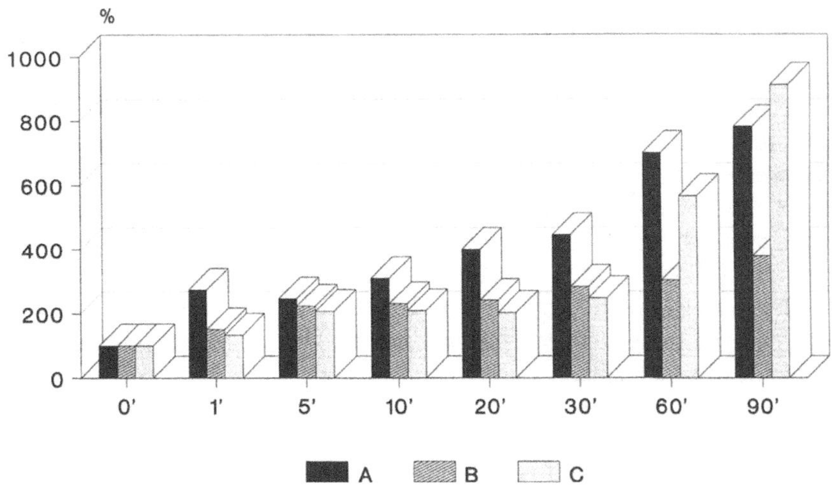

Fig. 8. FPA (fibrinopeptid A) vs. time.

Discussion

The oxygenators of the individual manufacturers behave completely differently with regard to the further factor XII induced pathway. Thus, oxygenation systems A and B show the following course: the α-fragment is formed to a greater degree whereas with oxygenator C, the rise of β-fragment is significantly marked, thus, activating the kallikrein-kinin system. This means that in vivo an increased drop in blood pressure is to be expected caused by the kallikrein rise with the use of oxygenator C. This can lead to a threatening situation especially in the case of the newborn and small children (3, 13).

The activation of FXII and the role played by the other contact phase proteins have been dealt with by us in the literature through earlier studies (2, 8). It is thought that when FXII (mol. wt. 80000) is bonded to negatively-charged surfaces an autoactivation then occurs causing the swift generation of α- and β-FXIIa and kallikrein. α-FXIIa is a two-chained active enzyme made of fragments bonded by disulphide connections with a mol. wt. of 57000 and 28000. The proteolytic dissociation of α-FXIIa generates an active enzyme with mol. wt. 28000 which first carried the name Hageman factor (FXIIf) and was later called β-factor XIIa. While α-FXIIa forms bonds at negatively charged surfaces, β-FXIIa does not. α- and β-FXIIa both activate PK whereby α-FXIIa is a much more effective activator of FXII than β-FXIIa. It was also possible to show that α-FXIIa and β-FXIIa activate other proenzymes including FVII, plasminogen and C1. Since KK is such a strong activator of surface-bonded FXII and since both α- and β-FXIIa convert PK to KK, there is a self-amplification with the explosive activation of FXII. The generation of FXII thus occurring does not only lead to further activity of FXII but also to the release of bradykinin from HMW-kininogen (6). Bradykinin increases the permeability of the vessels, causes hypotension, leads to contraction of the smooth muscles, causes pain, and releases tissue-plasminogen activator. KK further, converts plasminogen into plasmin, releases α- and β-factor XIIa from FXII, releases renin from prorenin, and stimulates the neutrophil granulocytes to begin chemotactic activity (8). The activation of factor XII also occurs at artificial surfaces particularly in ECC as we have already been able to show in previous model investigations. Such an activation also takes place at exposed collagenous connective tissue and at the damaged vascular wall. Endotoxin, for example, is a biological activator.

Depending on the heparin employed there is a significant activation of FXII. At the same time the pathway can be shown via the fragments α-factor XIIa and β-factor XIIa.

The kallikrein system plays an important role, its activation representing a measure of the reaction with negatively charged artificial surfaces. The inactivation of plasma kallikrein occurs via an irreversible complex formation with the C1-inactivator. The influence gained by the C1-inactivator with the plasma kallikrein inhibition can be seen clearly when the function of plasma kallikrein is observed. Two main functions are to be mentioned here: on the one hand, the formation of vasoactive bradykinin from HMW-kininogen and, on the other, the influence on the intrinsic part of coagulation through an activation of factor XIIa (Hageman factor).

Prekallikrein is the inactive preliminary stage of the plasma kallikrein and is converted to kallikrein through the surface-activated Hageman factor. The activation through the activated Hageman factor leads to a molecule bonded via a disulphide bridge and with a heavy chain of 52000 daltons and a light chain of 37000 or 42000 daltons. The light chain contains the activation center. On the other hand kallikrein can again activate factor XII in the sense of positive feedback.

Kallikrein can release bradykinin through proteolysis of HMW-kininogen. The effects of bradykinin are

- ▶ reduction in the peripheral resistance
- ▶ hypotension
- ▶ increase in vascular permeability
- ▶ hemoconcentration
- ▶ release of prostaglandins
- ▶ influence of vasotonus
- ▶ pain
- ▶ release of histamine from the mast cells of the lung
- ▶ increase in the cellular glucose intake in the sceletal muscle.

Since during extracorporeal circulation (ECC) the passage of the blood through the lung is cut off, there is not sufficient metabolization of bradykinin as the kininases are particularly located in the endothelial cells of the lung.

The kininase II (angiotensin converting enzyme) converts angiotensin I to angiotensin II. During ECC, the increasing amounts of kinins compete with angiotensin I for the kininase. As the affinity constant for kinins is higher, there is a drop in the angiotensin II concentration which again influences the vasotonus.

Kallikrein is an activator of plasminogen and can thus influence the fibrinolytic system. Further, there is a connection to the complement system since kallikrein can release C1-esterase via plasmin from its inactive preliminary stage. In addition kallikrein possesses chemotactic properties for neutrophil granulocytes and monocytes. C1-esterase inhibitor, alpha-2-macroglobulin, and antithrombin III are involved in the kallikrein inhibition. Further complex formation of the C1-inactivator with plasmin and thus an influence on fibrinolysis was observed. Through a surplus of plasmin this complex can be broken down into an inactive inhibitor with reduced molecular weight which not only can inhibit the C1-plasmin but also makes the reverse possible. In addition, however, an inhibitory effect of C1-inactivator on trypsin, though weak, was detectable.

Results of our investigations have shown that the heparin applied represents a decisive factor for possible postoperative lung complications after aortocoronary bypass operations. Thus, these results are to be viewed under the aspect Heparin: a risk factor? and with regard to possible subsequent lung complications that occur through damage to the endothelium.

According to Gallimore and Friberger the kallikrein inhibition mainly represents the capacity of C1-esterase inhibitor to inhibit plasma kallikrein. Alpha-2-macroglobulin seems to play an important role as quick inactivator for measuring the kallikrein inhibition. Therefore, possibly a masked intraoperative drop in alpha-2-macroglobulin must be assumed. Since this is the case, no important influence on the kallikrein inhibition can be attributed to alpha-2-macroglobulin. Experimental studies have shown that with the direct application of kallikrein to the plasma 57% of the C1-esterase inhibitor bonds with kallikrein, whereas with kallikrein, endogenously activated via negatively charged surfaces, only 16% bonds with alpha-2-macroglobulin and 82% with the C1-esterase inhibitor. The influence of alpha-2-macroglobulin on the kallikrein inhibition in in vivo studies should be rethought since it is probably negligibly slight with kallikrein produced via contact activation. However, with these inhibitors Harper et al. points out a temperature-dependent effect, whereby at low temperatures alpha-2-macroglobulin comes in the foreground. Despite hypothermia it was not possible to detect any relevant influence on the part of alpha-2-macroglobulin on kallikrein inhibition.

The results of the PMN elastase illustrate to what extent the granulocytes are damaged by different oxygenators, whereby in the course of recirculation it becomes clear how membrane-damaging the individual oxygenator are.

With the platelets the membrane-damaging effect becomes even more evident. This is measured via platelet factor 4 (PF4) or also via the platelet count (1, 19, 20). This means that the membrane-damaging effect is dependent on the oxygenator applied in each case. Since the damaged platelets act as secondary artificial surfaces, this effect is reinforced further and has an influence on the contact system.

Observing the behavior of the cellular components of the blood, the oxygenator system C shows the lowest degree of hemolysis as a measure of the destruction of erythrocytes (11). Platelet factor 4 (PF4), taken as a measure of damage to the platelets, rises significantly with oxygenators A and B already after 1 minute of recirculation (16). The latter oxygenators similar results are to be found as a measure of granulocyte damage, with a significant rise in the PMN elastase. Thus, the application of oxygenators A and B leads to a significantly increased damage to the corpuscular components of the blood, and in this context the behavior of the coagulation system is of interest. Here we observe similar behavior in oxygenators A and B to that of oxygenator C, whereby the latter is clearly inferior to the other two as can be seen in the significantly high TAT and FPA levels at the end of recirculation. The study shows that the individual oxygenator systems do partly differ; however, we cannot speak of a common tendency with regard to the investigated parameters. A differentiated weighing of the positive and negative criteria is, therefore, absolutely essential.

In summary it can be said that with regard to the quality, particularly of a pediatric oxygenator, this first depends significantly on the size of the artificial surface, including the heat exchanger for the extent of contact phase activation; second, it is essential to consider the damage of the cellular blood components; and third, the behavior of the coagulation system, particularly of TAT and FPA, is of great importance with respect to the formation of thrombosis and to restenosis.

In analogy to the clotting cascade, the activation of fibrinolysis can occur intrinsically or via an extrinsic path. The endogenous activation of fibrinolysis is closely connected to the contact activation of clotting. Besides activated factor XII, kallikrein and factor XIa are also able to activate plasminogen. The most important extrinsic activator is the tissue-type plasminogen activator (t-PA) which is released from the endothelial cells of the vascular wall. Urokinase is a further physiological activator.

Conclusion

With the introduction of membrane oxygenators in heart surgery, it was apparently not obvious just what problems this was to bring with it. The many and diverse questions with regard to contact of the blood with artificial surfaces at and between the artificial membranes have, up to today, not been adequately resolved and will, no doubt, continue to occupy our attention for a good deal of time to come. Within the framework of the present study, systems of pediatric oxygenators of different types were tested in a heart-lung model (HLM) developed by our group (A comparative study for adult oxygenators exists, showing other results). Our main focus of interest was on the proteins of the contact phase, on the one hand, and the extrinsic pathway and the cellular components of the blood during extracorporeal circulation (ECC), on the other. A further important aspect of the study was the behavior of the coagulation system.

With the study, it was our hope to demonstrate that the findings from the pathophysiology of the clotting system, contact phase, and fibrinolysis show that it is clinically of great relevance to demonstrate (such results) in the model system at artificial devices and to recognize necessarily corresponding changes. We also find this extremely necessary because nowadays we perform surgery on ever younger and ever older patients, both of whom are ill, and increasingly susceptable, dependent in terms of survival on an essential equilibrium and interaction of all organic systems.

References

1. Boldt J, Zickmann B, Czeke A, Herold C, Dapper F, Hempelmann G (1991) Blood conservation techniques and platelet function in cardiac surgery. Anaesthesiology 75:426–432
2. Colman RW (1995) Hemostatic complications of cardiopulmonary bypass. Am J Hematol 48:267–272
3. Colman RW, Schmaier AH (1997) Contact system: a vascular biology modulator with anticoagulant, profibrinolytic, antiadhesive, and proinflammatory attributes. Blood 90:3819–3843
4. Colman RW, Scott CF, Schmaier AH, Wachtfogel YT, Pixley RA, Edmunds LH Jr (1987) Initiation of blood coagulation at artificial surfaces. In: Leonard EF, Turrito VT, Vroman L (eds) Ann N Y Acad Sci 253–267
5. del Nido PJ, Armitage JM, Fricker FJ et al (1994) Extracorporeal membrane oxygenation support as a bridge to pediatric heart transplantation. Circulation 90:II66–II69
6. Egberg N, Gallimore MJ, Green K, Jacobsson J, Vesterqvist O, Wiman B (1988) Effects of plasma kallikrein and bradykinin infusions into pigs on plasma fibrinolytic variables and urinary excretion of thromboxane and prostacyclin metabolites. Fibrinolysis 2:101–106
7. el Habbal MH, Carter H, Smith LJ, Elliott MJ, Strobel S (1995) Neutrophil activation in paediatric extracorporeal circuits: effect of circulation and temperature variation. Cardiovasc Res 29:102–107
8. Fuhrer G, Gallimore MJ, Heller W, Hoffmeister HE (1990) F XII (Review). Blut 61:258–266
9. Groom RC, Akl BF, Albus R, Lefrak EA (1996) Pediatric cardiopulmonary bypass: a review of current practice. Int Anesthesiol Clin 34:141–163
10. Hamsten A (1993) The hemostatic system and coronary heart disease. Thromb Res 70:1–38
11. Harker LA (1986) Bleeding after cardiopulmonary bypass. N Engl J Med 314:1446–1447
12. Heller W, Wendel HP (1993) Clivarin and other LMWHs in an ex vivo cardiopulmonary bypass model. Studies on contact activation. Blood Coagul Fibrinolysis 4:45–54
13. Mammen EF (1990) Contact activation: The interaction of clotting, fibrinolytic, kinin and complement systems. Biomedical Progress 2:31–34
14. Nicolas F, Daniel JP, Bruniaux J, Serraf A, Lacour Gayet F, Planche C (1994) Conventional cardiopulmonary bypass in neonates. A physiological approach – 10 years of experience at Marie-Lannelongue Hospital. Perfusion 9:41–48
15. Plotz FB, van Oeveren W, Bartlett RH, Wildevuur CR (1993) Blood activation during neonatal extracorporeal life support. J Thorac Cardiovasc Surg 105:823–832
16. Rinder CS, Bohnert J, Rinder HM, Mitchell J, Ault K, Hillman R (1991) Platelet activation and aggregation during cardiopulmonary bypass. Anaesthesiology 75:388–393
17. Seghaye MC, Duchateau J, Grabitz RG et al (1994) Complement, leukocytes, and leukocyte elastase in full-term neonates undergoing cardiac operation. J Thorac Cardiovasc Surg 108:29–36

18. Sonntag J, Dahnert I, Stiller B, Hetzer R, Lange PE (1998) Complement and contact activation during cardiovascular operations in infants. Ann Thorac Surg 65:525–531
19. Stanford MF, Munoz PC, Vroman L (1983) Platelets adhere where flow has left fibrinogen on glass. Ann N Y Acad Sci 416:504–512
20. Wenger RK, Lukasiewicz H, Mikuta BS, Niewiarowski S, Edmunds LH (1989) Loss of platelet fibrinogen receptors during clinical cardiopulmonary bypass. J Thorac Cardiovasc Surg 97:235–239

Author's address:
Prof. Dr. W. Heller
Dr. H. P. Wendel
Abteilung für Thorax-, Herz- und Gefäßchirurgie
Eberhard-Karls-Universität Tübingen
Calwerstr. 7/1
D-72076 Tübingen
Germany

Material and circuit related bioincompatibility of cardiopulmonary bypass in cardiovascular surgery

S. Daniel
Boulogne, France

Introduction

This presentation is intended to cover the pathophysiology of cardiopulmonary bypass (CPB) (5, 6) linked to the bypass circuit and to the material or foreign surfaces interacting with the patient's blood and how those blood activators contribute to the deleterious consequences of CPB impacting the postoperative complications or morbidity. Other areas will be covered by other presenters.

In 1999, it is important to acknowledge that the pathophysiology or bioincompatibility of bypass is complex and multifactorial. See Fig. 1 for a picture of four major areas of blood activation potentially leading to post-operative complications.

- Material related.
- Circuit related, the mechanical forces generated within a non-endothelial, artificial circuit and a non-physiological flow environment (2, 4, 9, 10, 12).
- Surgery related, particularly but not exclusively related to the tissue injury, also drug therapy such as heparin and protamine or their formed complex and to the air-blood interface through the cardiotomy blood aspirations (7).
- Patient-related conditions more specifically related to his or her genetic background. It is now believed that the reason one patient may be more or less affected by the aggression of CPB is linked to his or her genetic heritage that will mediate the cytotoxic components generated during CPB in open heart surgery (the genetic factors are just starting to be better understood but will require a lot more work in order to elucidate the mechanisms) (13).

First let us focus on the interactions of the artificial or non-physiological surfaces and the patient's blood and what during CPB are some of the visible clinical effects not necessarily yet fully understood.

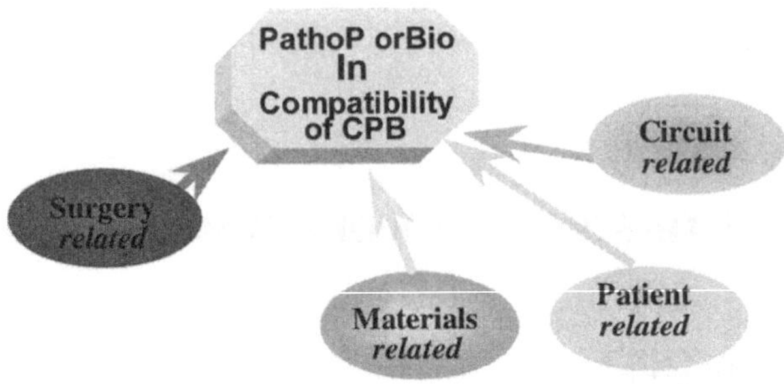

Fig. 1. Pathophysiology or bioincompatibility of CPB in 1999: complex and multifactorial.

Blood interactions with foreign, non-physiological surfaces like artificial materials

When blood and all its cellular and immunological components come in contact with foreign surfaces, the various patient defence mechanisms are recruited and activated. It is not as yet well established in which order those events take place (5, 6). What is known is that it is a dynamic process with most of the steps, once initiated, being irreversible.

- Initially there is a massive adsorption of proteins and particularly fibrinogen on the foreign surface. Either if the surface is hydrophobic or to a lesser degree if it is hydrophilic.
- As soon as the fibrinogen sticks to the non-physiological surface, all other activations that follow will contribute with various degrees to the formation or generation of the thrombus.
- The intrinsic plasma coagulation cascade is activated through the contact phase via four proteases: FXII, KK, HMWK, and FXI. This pathway leads to the formation of thrombin, fibrin and finally the thrombus.
- FXII and KK are then directly activating the neutrophils and monocytes contributing to the release of vasoactive and cytotoxic substances playing a role in the activation of the endothelium and the inflammatory response.
- The anaphylatoxins C3a and C5a are then activated via an alternate pathway. Both of these proteins are able to recruit and activate the leukocytes.
- The platelets then stick to the adhesive sites of the fibrinogen, through their glycoproteins GPIIb/GPIIIa (located on their outer membrane). Consequently, the platelets will adhere to others; they will aggregate and become activated.
- Finally, the activation of the platelets through their contact with fibrinogen will release alpha granules, GMP 140 or P selectin expressed on the outer membrane of the platelets and will recruit and further activate the leukocytes and more specifically the neutrophils and the monocytes. P selectin mediates the rolling of the leukocytes on the endothelium and platelet adhesion particularly to the neutrophils and monocytes which are considered to be the first step of the inflammation cascade of the whole body.

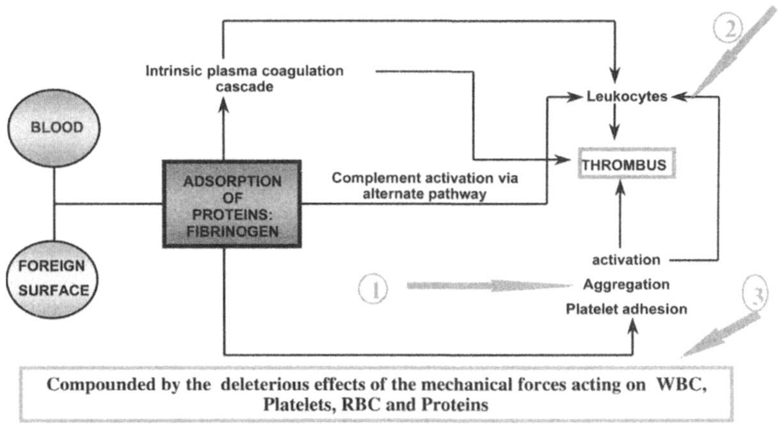

Fig. 2. Blood interactions with foreign, non-physiological surfaces, like today's artificial materials.

We are now able to review some manifestations of certain pathways that can be triggered during clinical CPB.

As shown in Fig. 2, we will first (arrow1) examine how the platelet activation under certain circumstances can manifest itself during CPB, then we will look at (arrow2) another manifestation most probably triggered by the humoral or immune defense mechanism that is far from being completely understood, and finally, we will put in perspective the role of the fluid dynamics or mechanical forces generated within the artificial bypass circuit and potentially leading to post-operative complications (arrow3). One must understand at this point that those deleterious effects are compounded by other blood activators such as air, drugs, oxygen levels, etc.

Oxygenator vasoconstriction or high pressure excursion (arrow 1)

This first clinical example illustrating the manifestation of blood interacting with foreign surfaces or artificial materials is linked to the platelets and have sometimes wrongly been reported as a malfunction of the oxygenator.

Figure 3 shows the end-view of an oxygenator hollow fiber bundle or membrane. Before the first passage of blood, right before the bypass is initiated, one can observe a clear or patent blood pathway with the inter-fiber space being at a maximum. The same observation can be made for a flat sheet membrane. At this time, if one is actually monitoring the inlet and oulet pressures of the oxygenator, they will translate on an analog graph as shown on Fig. 4, to the outlet pressure and pressure drop across the oxygenator remaining constant as a function of time (assuming the arterial blood flow is constant).

When bypass is then initiated, the patient's blood comes in contact with a large foreign surface area, the fibrinogen is adsorbed, and some platelets

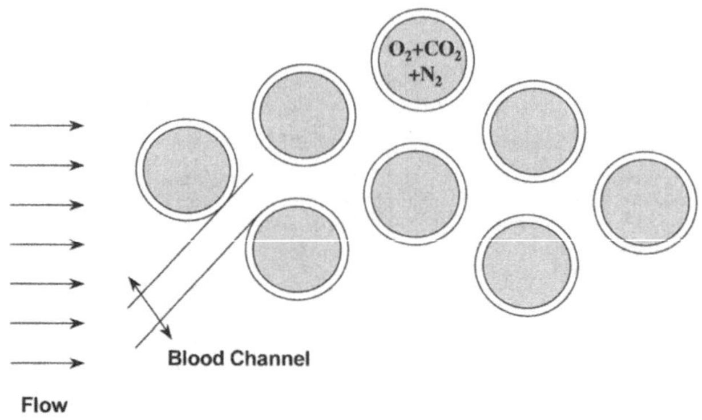

Fig. 3. End-view of oxygenator hollow fibers during priming, but before bypass.

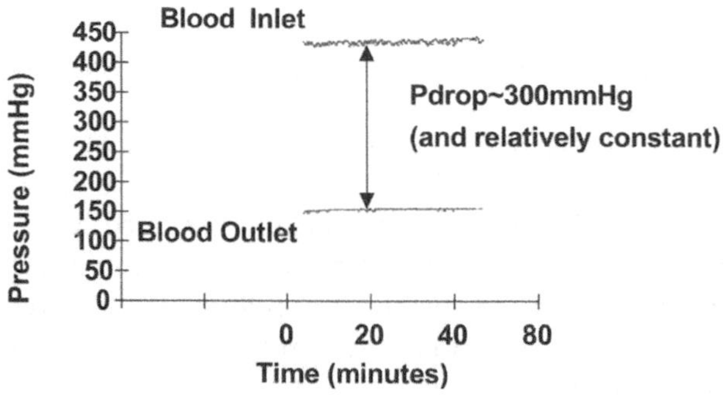

Fig. 4. Normal pressure drop across an oxygenator.

stick to the hollow fibers forming a microlayer of fibrinogen, combined with platelets modifying or reducing the fiber inter-space or the width of the blood pathway (see Fig. 5) (11). This occurrence will result in an increase of the flow resistance as shown in Fig. 6 with several consequences:

- The pressure drop across the oxygenator is increased independently of the blood temperature, viscosity or hemodilution.
- The inlet pressure is increased beyond the normal expected levels and may alarm or even panic an untrained perfusionist.

This high excursion pressure observed at the inlet of the oxygenator with an increase in pressure drop across the oxygenator has been reproduced using an in vitro model. The graphs shown in Figs. 4 and 6 correspond to the results from the in vitro model reproducing the phenomena experienced under certain circumstances with certain patients in clinical CPB.

However, we now know that a certain sensitive patient population exists accounting for approximately 4% of the total population exhibiting this rather abnormal *transient high excursion pressure.* This transient effect (assuming

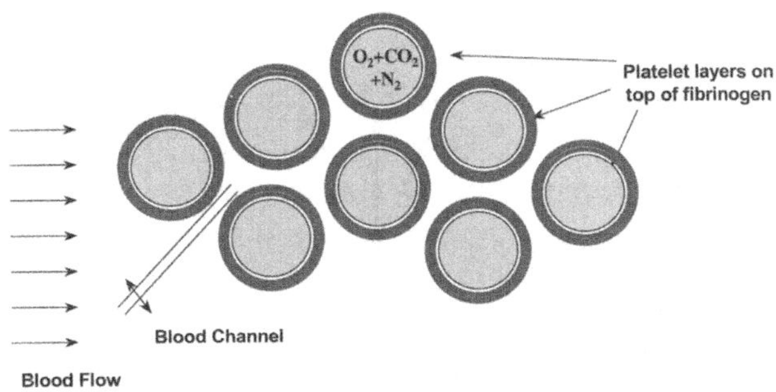

Fig. 5. End-view of oxygenator hollow fibers 10–15 min into bypass.

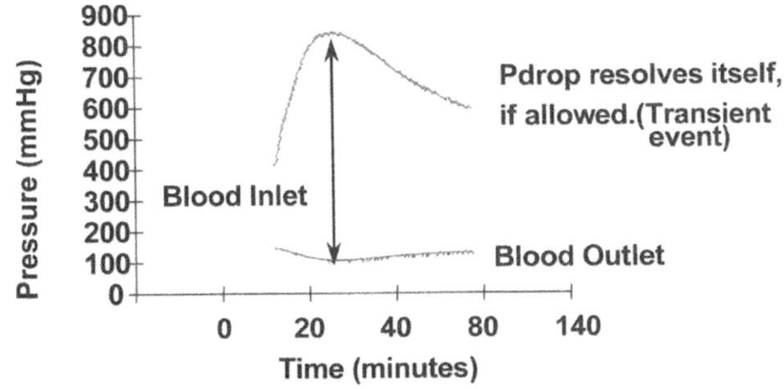

Fig. 6. Abnormal pressure excursion or pressure drop across any oxygenator and seen on less than 4% of CPB.

one is actually confronted with a patient with abnormal or excessive reaction to foreign material) should disappear after several minutes into bypass.

Influence of the material and related cellular and immune activations on the endothelium function (arrow 2)

This second manifestation may be linking the material with the endothelium. However, this phenomena is far from being completely understood and several hypotheses have been formulated (1, 3, 8, 11, 14, 16).

In plasmapheresis similar to CPB, a transient arterial pressure drop (see Fig. 7) or hypotension induced by the contact of the patient's blood with foreign surfaces of the plasmapheresis or cardiac artificial bypass circuits have been observed (see Fig. 7) (14, 15).

The only marked difference with CPB is the time of occurrence as the hypotension in plasmapheresis occurs late after the initiation of the treatment as opposed to CPB. From the clinical study (15) published in Japan, they have apparently attributed this pressure fall to the activation of the complement through the alternate pathway with anaphylatoxine C3a and C5a. The other clinical study (14) performed by Fraze Rubens from Ottawa, Canada

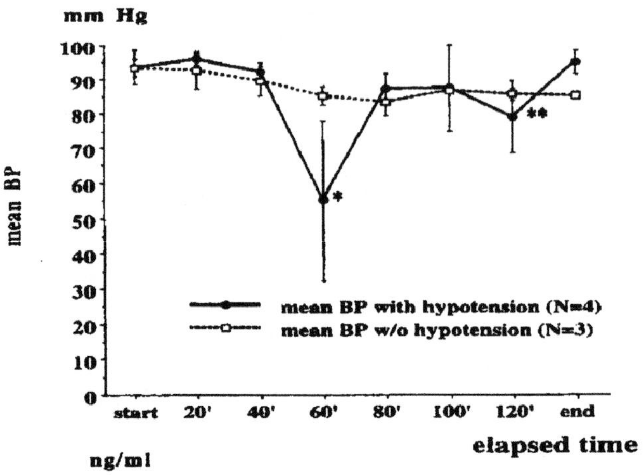

Fig. 7. Transient hypotension during plasmapheresis (from (15)).

compared randomly a cohort of 17 patients treated with a conventional untreated bypass circuit and a cohort of 17 patients treated with a more biocompatible (surface modification additives) surface from tip to tip, not just the oxygenator. The conditions as described in the paper are exactly the same: the circuit is primed with crystalloid and is performed in normothermia on patients with uncomplicated coronary bypass, the aspirated blood from the surgical field is not mixed nor retransfused with the patient's systemic blood.

As observed (Fig. 8) at the initiation of bypass, a transient arterial radial pressure drop or hypotension of 100% of the untreated bypass circuit population. The first general reaction is to explain this transient event as being due to the change of viscosity linked to hemodilution. This is correct but can only account for 3 to 5 mmHg and not for more than 30 mmHg as shown on the graph. Consequently it must be due to more than the viscosity as the conditions are the same for the other SMA population. However, 100% of the SMA population treated with a more biocompatible material comprising the total bypass circuit does not exhibit this hemodynamic pressure effect. One may also think that it may be a physiological reaction (vaso-vagal reflex), but then why would this be only found in one population (not the SMA). The only difference being the quality of the foreign surface in contact with the patient's blood.

Therefore, we may at this point hypothesize that this phenomena is a transient vasodilation or a fluid shift from the intravascular bed to the extravascular interstial space but in all cases linked to an endothelium response. Assuming it is a *vasodilatation* of the endothelium, what can induce this response?

- Generation of bradykinin linked to the contact phase activation? Will the effect on the radial pressure be so fast?

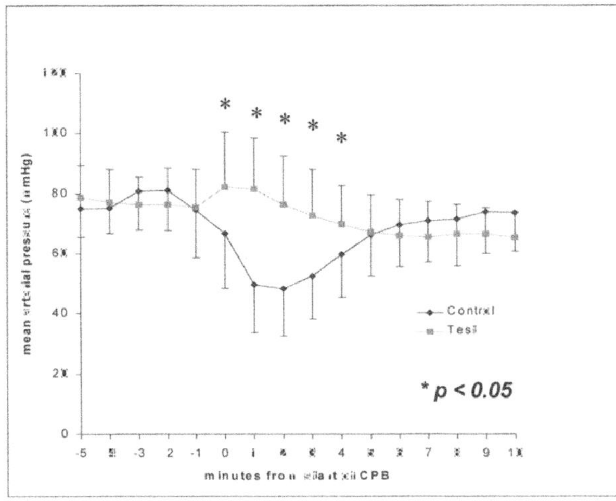

Fig. 8. Radial artery mean blood pressure in mmHg at initiation of CPB (from (14)).

- Activation of the complement C3a and C5a with induction of histamine? We know that the response is slow.
- Activation of certain cellular immune complexes promoting the release of nitric oxyde (NO) by the endothelium?

Assuming it is *a fluid shift*, what can induce this response?

- Massive change of the endothelium permeability linked to elastase, TNF from leukocytes, and P selectin from platelets. We know that those components entrain a very fast response at the endothelium level. However can the permeability change alone explain a drop of more than 30 mmHg?

We need to investigate further to better understand how clinically those manifestations really impact the patient condition postoperatively and what the actual mechanisms are.

Flow dynamics or mechanical forces and the impairments of the formed components of blood and proteins (arrow 3)

In 1994 Hellum and Hardwick were studying in vitro a viscosity meter the response of the formed element of blood to mechanical stresses such as shear stress. They demonstrated at this time very clearly and elegantly that the mechanical stresses are even more prominent in term of deleterious effects than the blood interacting with foreign or artificial surfaces (2, 4, 9, 10, 12). In summary they show that the leukocytes are activated at a shear stress level of more than 75 dynes per square centimeter. The platelets are activated above 100 dynes/cm^2. However, the red cells or erythrocytes can withstand

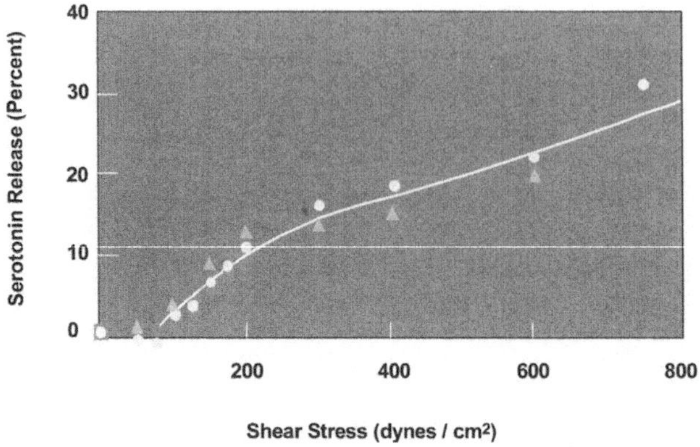

Fig. 9. Release of serotonin by platelets as a function of shear stress. In vitro contitions: t=5 min; 3 s/v values=■ 141 cm^{-1}, ● 87, ▲ 57 (from 3)).

rather high shear stress as no hemolysis is induced at shear stress below 2000 dynes/cm^2. As a point of clarification, within an artificial cardio-pulmonary bypass circuit, the generated shear stress is a function of the geometry or the dimension design characteristics of the bypass circuit and also the blood flow conditions controlled by the arterial blood pump.

On the graph shown as an example in Fig. 9, one can see the platelets being activated above 100 dynes/cm^2. However what is equally important is the fact that the study by Hellum and Hardwick was performed at three different surface areas of foreign surface in contact with blood. They have shown that the platelet activation is virtually nonmaterial dependent with the most dominant source of activation being the shear stress and not the foreign nature of the material.

Conclusion

In cardiopulmonary bypass, the platelets are certainly the most damaged blood components (Fig. 10). Their role in the first step of the inflammatory reactions along with the leukocytes, mediated by the mechanical forces and the foreign surfaces most certainly affect the endothelium function through mechanisms apparently not yet fully understood. In any event, this perturbed important function must impact the postoperative patient outcome. The "how" remains to be further studied clinically.

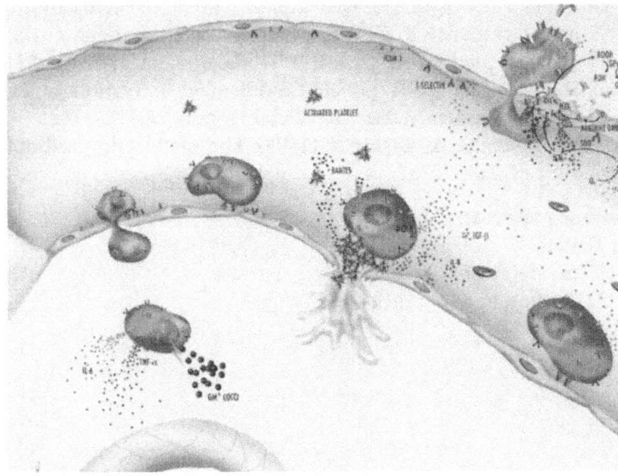

Fig. 10. Perturbed and damaged endothelium function by the couple platelets, leukocytes.

References

1. Asimakopoulos G, Taylor K (1998) Effects of cardiopulmonary bypass on leukocytes and endothelial adhesion molecules. Ann Thorac Surg 66:2135–2144
2. Barstad RM, Roald HE, Cui Y, Turitto VT, Sakariassen KS (1994) A perfusion chamber developed to investigate thrombus formation and shear profiles in flowing native human blood at the apex of well-defined stenoses. Arteriosclerosis Tromo 14:1984–1991
3. Bonomini M, Settefrati N (1999) Interactions between platelets and leukocytes during hemodialysis. Artificial Organs (23)1:23–28
4. Butler J, Westaby S (1992) Platelet responses to cardiopulmonary bypass (assessment by a shear stress activation technique). Oxford J Cardiovasc Surg 33:33–37
5. Daniel S (1996) Review of the multifactorial aspects of BioInCompatibility in CPB. Perfusion 11:246–255
6. Daniel S Is the artificial, foreign surface the single culprit for the post-operative complications of CPB? How can a new surface modification technology ameliorate the bioIncompatibility of to day's CPB. (In preparation)
7. de Haan J, Boonstra PW, Monnink SHJ, Ebels T, van Oeveren W (1995) Retransfusion of suctioned blood during cardiopulmonary bypass impairs hemostasis. Ann Thorac Surg 59:901–907
8. Meinrad P, Gawaz H, Gurland J (1999) Platelet-leukocytes aggregates during hemodyalysis. Effects of membrane type. Artificial Organs (23)1:29–36
9. Hellum JD (1993) Whitaker Lecture: Biorheology in thrombosis research. Ann Biomed Eng 22:445–455
10. Hellum JD, Hardwick RA (1994) Response of platelets to shear stress. In: Gross DR, Hwang NHC (eds) The Rheology of Blood, Blood Vessels and Associated Tissues. Rockville, MD: Sijthoff and Noordhoff pp 160–183
11. Inui K, Shiono S (1998) Aprotin reduces the expression of P selectin on the surface of platelet and leukocytes-platelets conjugates. Artificial Organs 22(12):1018–1022
12. Podias A, Groth Th, Missirlis Y (1994) The effect of shear stress on the adhesion/activation of human platelets in flow through a closed loop polymeric tubular system. J Biomater Sci polymer 6:399–410
13. Rochette L Perspectives dans la protection myocardique: originalités théoriques. Faculté de médecine et de pharmacie, Dijon, France

14. Rubens FD et al (1998) Circuits with surface modifying additives alter the hemodynamic response to CPB in cardiac surgical patient. Ottawa, Canada. Abstract submitted and accepted to the 1998 EACTS meeting in Brussels, Belgium
15. Shiga Y, Itoyama Y (1998) Complement activation as a cause of transient hypotension during plasmapheresis. Artificial Organs 22:112–116
16. Weerasinghe A, Taylor K (1998) The platelet in cardiopulmonary bypass. Ann Thorac Surg 66:2145–2152

Author's address:
S. Daniel
110 Rue de Paris
F-92100 Boulogne, France

Alterations of the hemostaseologic system under extracorporeal conditions

H. Trobisch
Institute of Hematology and Transfusion Medicine, Duisburg, Germany

Extracorporeal perfusion exposes blood to large surface areas composed of synthetic polymers and lacking endothelial cells, and the effects of these factors on blood elements produce an absolute requirement for heparin to prevent clotting.

During extracorporeal perfusion for cardiac surgery, autologous blood is routinely diluted to a hematocrit of about 25% by priming the extracorporeal circuit with nonblood crystalloid solutions. A heparin dose of 3 mg/kg is usually adequate to prevent fibrin formation during cardiopulmonary bypass (CPB).

The changes in blood composition during extracorporeal perfusion are multiple. Some blood elements are activated and consumed; others are destroyed; some are not altered. Vasoactive substances and microemboli are produced (2).

Blood contact with artificial surfaces directly activates Factor XII and platelets. Cleavage of FXII on synthetic surfaces in the presence of the other primary contact proteins, e.g., Factor XI, prekallikrein, and high molecular weight kininogen initiates the intrinsic coagulation system by generating Factor XIa. Plasmin, kallikrein, and bradykinin are also generated. Factor XII fragments stimulate C1 – the first component of complement – and activate C3 and C5 by the classical complement pathway. The activation peptides of these complement factors C3a and C5a promote vasodilatation and hypotension (1).

Activation of blood coagulation depends on the type of oxygenator used. Negatively charged artificial surfaces can activate Factor XII directly. In time, it will activate the intrinsic coagulation cascade which leads to thrombin and fibrin formation. The increase of the concentrations of prothrombin fragment 1.2 and TAT complex shows the extent of activation. But breakdown of coagulation like in the case of DIC are very seldom. Therefore, there is every reason to believe that activation of coagulation is compensated during CPB by the physiologic inhibitors within the oxygenator, especially by the antithrombin-heparin complex. Carrying off of significant amounts of activated coagulation factors like thrombin or FXa within the circulation is unlikely.

As I pointed out, activation will be triggered by FXIIa and not by FVIIa, for this activated clotting factor could not be detected during CPB. On the other hand, it may be possible that this important cofactor of thromboplastin is rapidly inactivated by the tissue factor pathway inhibitor.

The amount of fibrin clots and macroaggregates formed within the oxygenator will be filtered out, so that only microaggregates of fibrin or platelets will be embolized into the patient. The embolization of microfibrin clots can activate the fibrinolytic system which will degrade them rapidly. Otherwise, these aggregates will be phagocytized by the RHS.

During CPB, platelet number and function decrease. The decline in platelet number is largely due to dilution, but adhesion to surfaces and formation of aggregates also contribute to this. The dysfunction of platelets is the most common hemostatic defect caused by CPB. Two reasons have been described. First, platelets become activated by contact with the artificial surfaces in the oxygenator. In addition, plasmin, ADP, heparin, and thrombin all activate platelets and thus the contents of α-granules are released. Platelets now develop a reduced response to agonists like ADP, collagen, and epinephrin in vitro. An acquired storage pool disease is the consequence – the so-called exhausted platelet syndrome. Furthermore, specific α-granule proteins were exposed on the surface of the platelets mainly p-selectin. Activated mononuclear cells had been shown to bind p-selectin with the formation of platelet-monocyte aggregates. These cellular aggregates can perhaps promote damage to the pulmonary microcirculation.

A second platelet function defect is caused by physical damage to platelet membranes during extracorporeal circulation. Platelets transient stick to the surfaces of the oxygenator, which damages membrane glycoproteins with receptor function. The mean number of fibrinogen and adrenergic receptors per circulating platelet decreases and platelet membrane fragments appear in the circulation. Hypothermia may accelerate this platelet function defect.

Electron micrographs of the circuit after use show a heterogenous population of platelets including intact activated platelets, partially and completely degranulated platelets, and platelet ghosts. The end result is an increase in postperfusion bleeding times and reduced platelet function and survival.

During CPB a short-lived activation of fibrinolysis may occur. Increased concentrations of tPA – released from endothelial cells during CPB – and a moderate fall in α-2-antiplasmin can be observed, but there are no signs of a systemic intravascular activation of the fibrinolytic system.

The concentration of fibrinogen falls only to the expected level of hemodilution and the concentration of fibrinogen split products is not markedly elevated. Nevertheless, secondary fibrinolysis is brisk due to the lysis of thrombi formed in the oxygenator and the surgical field. This is evidenced by a gradual increase in D-dimer concentration throughout CPB and several hours thereafter.

Clinical manifestations

Excessive and persistent bleeding from the chest tubes and wound sites is a common problem in the immediate postoperative period in cardiac surgery patients. The hourly volume of blood that drains from the chest tubes is an excellent indicator of the magnitude of bleeding, which frequently exceeds several hundred milliliters per hour. Oozing of blood from venipuncture sites or other areas of trauma suggests a systemic defect of hemostasis.

Laboratory tests

Preoperative screening tests in cardiac surgery patients are seldom predictive of postoperative bleeding, except for inborn errors of coagulation like v. Willebrands disease or hemophilia. The importance of inborn coagulation defects predisposing to thromboembolism – such as FV-Leiden and prothrombin mutation G20210A – is not known for CPB up to now. However, the bleeding time can be of use when it is obtained following the cessation of CPB.

Nearly all laboratory tests of coagulation are abnormal during and immediately following CPB because of hemodilution, the use of heparin, absorption of coagulation factors onto artificial surfaces, and platelet defects induced by the oxygenator. However, platelet counts are lower than predicted and platelet-specific membrane receptors like p-selectin are elevated; platelet-specific proteins like β-thromboglobulin are elevated, which suggests platelet activation. TAT-complex, D-dimer, and fibrinopeptide A are all elevated, but α-2-antiplasmin is decreased during CPB.

Laboratory tests should be obtained in cardiac surgery patients with postoperative bleeding and should include PT, PTT, fibrinogen, factor XIII, bleeding time (surgicut), and platelet count. Perhaps aggregation studies are indicated, if platelet count is subnormal and bleeding persists. The determination of heparin concentration is indicated if PTT and thrombin time are unclottable. In addition, fibrin monomer, D-dimer, and a fibrinolytic screening test may be of value. These tests are used to identify defects in coagulation, platelet function, and fibrinolysis, and as guides to clotting factor or platelet replacement therapy.

Other hemostatic problems relative to cardiac surgery

HAT2 syndrome

The use of unfractionated heparin during CPB and anticoagulant therapy with UFH may cause 7 to 14 days after CPB the heparin-associated thrombocytopenia type 2. IgG antibodies directed against the heparin platelet factor 4 complex – formed during heparin therapy – will aggregate and activate the majority of the circulating platelets. Multi-organ failure and severe bleeding will be the result.

Protamine toxicity

Some patients with diabetes mellitus who are treated with NPH insulin may develop IgG, IgA or IgE antibodies against protamine. When protamine is given to neutralize the heparin used for CPB, sensitized patients can suddenly develop pulmonary hypertension, hypoxia, and occasionally overwhelming DIC.

References

1. Khuri SF et al (1992) Hematologic changes during and after cardiopulmonary bypass and their relationship to the bleeding time and nonsurgical blood loss. J Thorac Cardiovasc Surg 104:94
2. Woodman RC, Harker LA (1990) Bleeding complications associated with cardiopulmonary bypass. Blood 76:1680

Author's address:
Prof. Dr. med. H. Trobisch
Fachlaboratorium für Hämatologie
Königstraße 53
D-47051 Duisburg
Germany

The systemic inflammatory response and myocardial injury during extracorporeal circulation

S. M. Wildhirt, C. Schulze, and B. Reichart
Department of Cardiac Surgery, Ludwig-Maximilians University, Munich, Germany

Introduction

Optimal myocardial protection remains a major concern in clinical cardiac surgery. The introduction of extracorporeal circulation and hypothermic cardioplegic arrest many years ago enabled the surgeon to perform cardiac surgery on the arrested heart and under safe conditions.

However, ischemia and reperfusion even under improved cardioprotection and hypothermia leads to activation of the systemic inflammatory response, considerable myocardial damage and is associated with substantial postoperative morbidity. In this regard, several attempts have been made to improve cardioprotection by modification of cardioplegic solutions, by providing extracorporeal circuits and oxygenators with precoated surfaces for enhanced protection of circulating blood cells or by pharmacological modification of the reperfusate (2, 4), and reperfusion induced injury is mediated by various mechanisms. These include increased adhesion of leukocytes to the endothelium contributing to "no reflow", generation of oxygen-derived free radicals with subsequent peroxidation of cellular structures and excessive increase of intracellular Ca^{++} which results in reversible and/or irreversible malfunction of the contractile apparatus.

One key element in the cascade of ischemia/reperfusion-induced injury is the activation of the vascular endothelium as the primary target for circulating blood cells and cytokines. Endothelial cell activation leads to an altered production of vasoactive mediators including nitric oxide, endothelin, and cytokines subsequently resulting in endothelial dysfunction. Impaired endothelial function leads to a pro-thrombotic state of the vasculature due to increased adhesion of activated platelets and neutrophils. In addition, impaired availability of endothelium-derived nitric oxide and activation of the endothelin system results in an enhanced vasoconstrictor tone and impaired regulation of organ blood flow (Fig. 1).

The present report summarizes recent findings related to the systemic pro-inflammatory response during CPB with special focus on the TNF system. In addition, we will discuss the potential role of two important vasoactive mediators, nitric oxide and endothelin, and the role of cell adhesion molecules on vascular function following CPB. Moreover, the potential con-

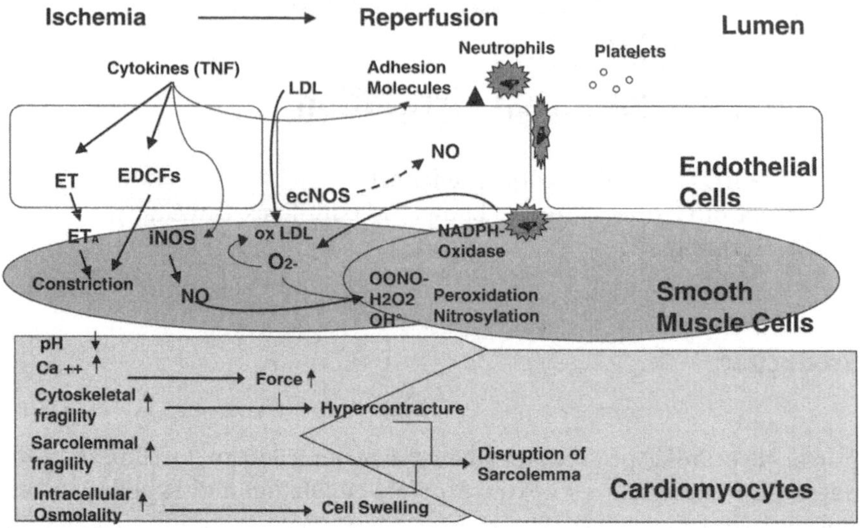

Fig. 1. A variety of factors contributing to ischemia/reperfusion (I/R)-induced injury during and following cardiopulmonary bypass (CPB). The immediate response to I/R includes changes in intracellular pH and calcium concentration, which increases intracellular force. This leads in the presence of increased cytoskeletal and sarcolemmal fragility to hypercontracture. In addition, an increase in intracellular osmolality and subsequent cell swelling results in disruption of the sarcolemma and cell death. Pro-inflammatory mediators are activated following I/R including cytokines. This results in the released and production of a variety of mediators contributing to impairment of cell and organ function. TNF-α mediates the expression of cell adhesion molecules on endothelial cells contributing to enhanced adhesion of platelets and neutrophils. In addition, TNF-α mediates the release of vasoconstricting factors such as endothelin but also activates inducible nitric oxide synthase (iNOS). The latter results in increased nitric oxide (NO) production which contributes to increased formation of oxygen radicals such as peroxynitrite ($ONOO^-$); it contributes to peroxidation and nitrosylation of cellular structures. In addition, ischemia results in increased formation of superoxide (O_2^-) particularly by activation of the NADPH-oxidase in infiltrating neutrophils, which significantly impairs endothelium-dependent vasomotor function by scavenging endothelium-derived NO.

tribution of CPB to oxyradical-mediated lipid peroxidation and myocardial cell damage will be outlined.

Cardiopulmonary bypass and activation of the TNF-α system

Cytokines are immunomodulators and signaling molecules involved in acute phase reactions. Various pathophysiologic conditions including ischemia/reperfusion (I/R), allograft rejection, heart failure, infectious diseases, sepsis, and CPB trigger their activation. It has been shown that after CPB the upregulation of these cytokines are associated with impaired myocardial contractility. It has been demonstrated that for example tumor necrosis factor α (TNF-α) exerts direct negative inotropic effects on the heart. However, TNF-α also enhances the activities of multiple mediators such as endothelin (ET) and nitric oxide synthase (NOS), the latter resulting in increased nitric oxide (NO) production; it also regulates the expression of adhesion molecules (P-selectin, ICAM-1) (Fig. 1). In addition, TNF-α is involved in induction of programmed cell death (apoptosis) (6, 14).

Apoptosis occurs under acute and chronic conditions such as after myocardial infarction or in the development of heart failure. Cardiac myocytes that undergo apoptotic cell death maintain their cell membrane integrity; therefore, apoptotic myocytes do not release creatine kinase and retain their ability to exclude dyes such as trypan blue. Indeed, it has been suggested that the degree on myocyte death by apoptosis during myocardial infarction may be underestimated. Moreover, apoptotic myocytes retain their contractile response after stimulation with calcium ionophores due to the maintenance of the myofilament responsiveness, whereas necrotic cells are already maximally contracted.

In addition, TNF-α exhibits a positive feedback induction of itself thereby further activating the pro-inflammatory response after the initial stimulus. TNF-α mediates the effects via two specific receptors (TNF-Rp1 and -Rp2) present on endothelial and smooth muscle cells, cardiomyocytes and other cell types such as macrophages. The negative inotropic effects of TNF-α are mediated by at least two different pathways. The NO-independent pathway involves the production of sphingosine from ceramide resulting in immediate changes in intracellular Ca^{++} transients. The negative inotropic effects are observed within minutes after TNF exposure (Fig. 2) (13). In contrast, the NO-dependent pathway requires de-novo synthesis of iNOS within inflammatory cells and cardiac myocytes. This is mediated by the activation of the nuclear transcription factor κB (NF-κB) which translocates into the cell nucleus. The enhanced NO production by increased iNOS activation decreases myofilament calcium sensitivity resulting in contractile dysfunction. This pathway is at least in part responsible for the delayed (hours/days) but sustained contractile dysfunction observed upon TNF activation (Fig. 2) (5).

Clinical examples of myocardial I/R-induced TNF-α release include myocardial infarction, angioplasty, and CPB. In particular during CPB it has been suggested that the heart is the primary source for enhanced TNF-α release as the concentration of the cytokine was significantly higher when compared to aortic plasma levels. Immunohistochemical analysis showed that TNF-α was predominately localized in myocytes and infiltrating mononuclear cells. These observations further support the notion that a therapeutic anti-TNF-α strategy may be a useful adjunct to cold cardioplegia during CPB.

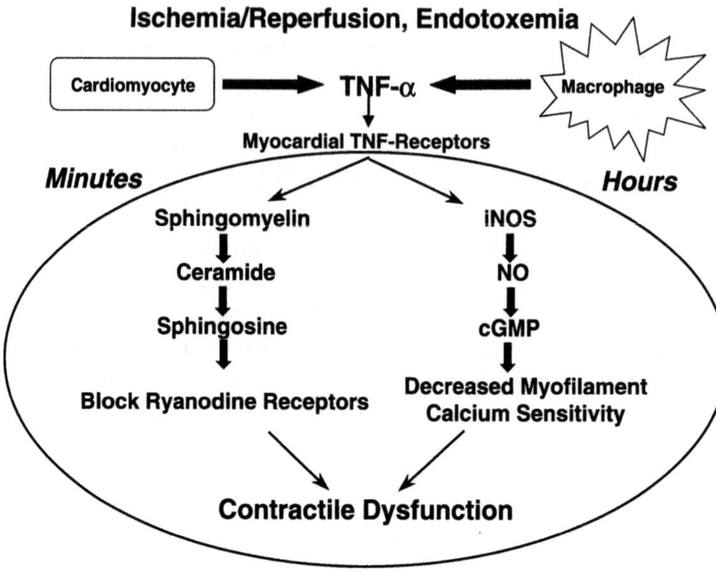

Fig. 2. TNF-α mediates its myocardial depressant effects via two specific receptors. TNF-α binding results in rapid release and production of sphingosine through sphingomyelin metabolism. Sphingosine is known to inhibit the ryanodine receptor, which results in inhibition of calcium-induced calcium release and cardiac contractile force. TNF-α also induces nitric oxide synthase (iNOS) resulting in delayed enhanced nitric oxide (NO) production. NO decreases myofilament sensitivity to cytosolic calcium and inhibits the β-adrenergic response thereby reducing contractility. These events occur within hours to days after ischemia/reperfusion or during endotoxemia.

Nitric oxide (NO) and endothelin during extracorporeal circulation

Nitric oxide

Nitric oxide is a potent vasodilator and free radical gas. Under physiologic conditions it is produced from a constitutive nitric oxide synthase in endothelial cells (ecNOS) in response to shear stress, pulsatile stretching of the vascular wall, and other stimuli such as thrombin, ATP, acetylcholine, serotonin or hypoxia (Fig. 3). ecNOS produces nanomolar concentrations if NO results not only in vasorelaxation but also inhibits adhesion of platelets and neutrophils to the endothelial cell layer. NO-dependent vasodilatation is mediated by cGMP through the activation of a soluble guanylate cyclase (sGC). cGMP activates a dependent protein kinase with subsequent extrusion if intracellular calcium via activation of a member-associated calcium/magnesium adenosine triphosphate pump. Continuous NO release by endothelial cells creates an active vasodilatory state responsible for homeostatic control of blood pressure and blood flow (12).

High amounts of NO (micromolar range) produced by the inducible NOS isoform (iNOS) have been shown to be responsible for a variety of pathophysiologic events that occur during acute inflammatory responses including

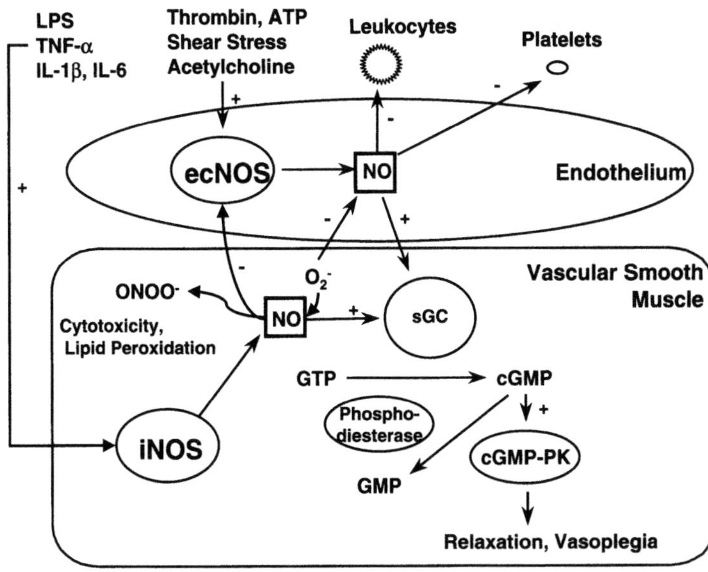

Fig. 3. The subcellular signal transduction pathway of nitric oxide (NO) is shown. NO is generated by different isozymes (NOS). The constitutive, endothelium-derived NOS (ecNOS) is active in endothelial cells and releases basal amounts of NO due to the conversion of the semi-essential amino acid L-arginine to L-citrulline in the presence of molecular oxygen. NO rapidly diffuses intraluminal or contraluminal where it acts by activation of the second messenge soluble guanylate cyclase; it converts guanosine monophosphate (GMP) into cyclic GMP (cGMP). cGMP activates a dependent proteinkinase, which leads to vascular smooth muscle relaxation due to changes in intracellular Ca^{2+}. NO also inhibits platelet and leukocyte adherence to endothelial cells. Under pathological conditions, stimuli such as TNF-α, IL-1β, IL-6, and LPS activate an inducible nitric oxide synthase (iNOS) in various cell types including vascular smooth muscle cells. High amounts of nitric oxide derived from this isozyme may result in peroxynitrite formation, which leads to cytotoxic effects on adjacent cells. In addition high amounts of cGMP may lead to vasoplegia due to an impaired response of vascular smooth muscle cells to β-adrenergic stimuli.

reduction of the systemic vascular resistance, hypotension, myocardial contractile dysfunction, and oxyradical mediated tissue damage. Under conditions of oxidative stress such as after cardiopulmonary bypass (CPB), NO may rapidly bind to superoxide (O_2^-) thereby forming peroxynitrite ($ONOO^-$) and hydroxyl radical ($^\bullet OH$), a powerful, highly reactive radical. Peroxynitrite nitrates and hydroxylates aromatic amino acids. The reaction product nitrotyrosine accounts as a marker for NO-mediated tissue damage. iNOS derived NO not only mediates direct detrimental effects but also inhibits endothelial-derived NO by a) increased scavenging of NO by superoxide and peroxynitrite, b) by induction of an isoform switch, i.e., inhibition of ecNOS expression by increased iNOS activation which results in endothelial dysfunction with a subsequent increase of cellular adhesion and impairment of blood flow regulation (1, 7).

Moreover, during systemic inflammation activated polymorphonuclear cells (PMN) are known to be potent sources of iNOS-derived NO. Depending on the redox state of the adjacent cell, PMN- and macrophage-derived NO may contribute to cellular injury and endothelial activation. In addition, increased iNOS activity in circulating blood cells such as platelets and neutrophils promotes a NO-mediated pro-thrombotic state of the vasculature. In this regard, CPB is associated with a systemic activation of the endothelium and may be associated with a significant reduction of endothelial NO production or its enhanced scavenging by oxyradicals such as superoxide. In this regard, it has been demonstrated that CPB decreased exhaled nitric oxide production suggesting that pulmonary vascular NO production was attenuated or scavenged which may be indicative for post-pump pulmonary hypertension often observed in these patients. However, reduced bioactive endothelium-derived NO may further induce NOS in the underlying smooth muscle cells contributing to a reduction of ventricular function and impaired coronary blood flow regulation to demand. Indeed, several authors have demonstrated a close relationship between post-bypass left ventricular dysfunction and increased iNOS-derived nitric oxide production (17, 18, 20). They reported deleterious effects on left ventricular function after administration of L-arginine, the substrate for the nitric oxide synthases. In addition, our own laboratory demonstrated that isoform-selective inhibition of increased NO production results in improvement of left ventricular systolic and diastolic function and reduction of infarct size. It also reduced the amount of infiltrating inflammatory cells within the reperfused myocardium and improved endothelium-dependent vasomotor function of the coronary circulation (21). Despite the concentration-dependent action of NO on cellular function, the redox state of the neighboring cells may also be responsible for the action of NO on cellular structures. A recent investigation from our laboratory showed that CPB for CABG resulted in significantly higher nitrite levels within 24–48 h after surgery when compared to off-pump surgery for coronary revascularization. In addition, systemic and myocardial malondialdehyde (MDA) levels, an indicator for lipid peroxydation, were significantly elevated during this time period; this suggests that enhanced NO production following CPB is associated with radical mediated tissue damage. Therefore, reduction of oxygen tension to maintain normoxic conditions may be of major therapeutic importance to prevent massive NO-mediated oxyradical formation during reperfusion.

Endothelin-1

Endothelin-1 (ET-1) is the most powerful endogenous vasoconstrictor known to date. This small peptide (23 amino acid sequence) is produced primarily in endothelial cells but is also expressed in smooth muscle cells. The final step to form the bioactive peptide is the proteolytic degradation of big-endothelin. ET-1 binds to two distinct receptors, ET-A and ET-B. The potent vasoconstrictor effect of ET-1 is mediated mainly by the ET-A receptor. As shown in Fig. 4, activation of the ET-A receptor results in an increase in phospholipase A which leads to the formation of inositol 1,4,5-triphosphate and diacylglycerol. The former is responsible for smooth muscle cell contrac-

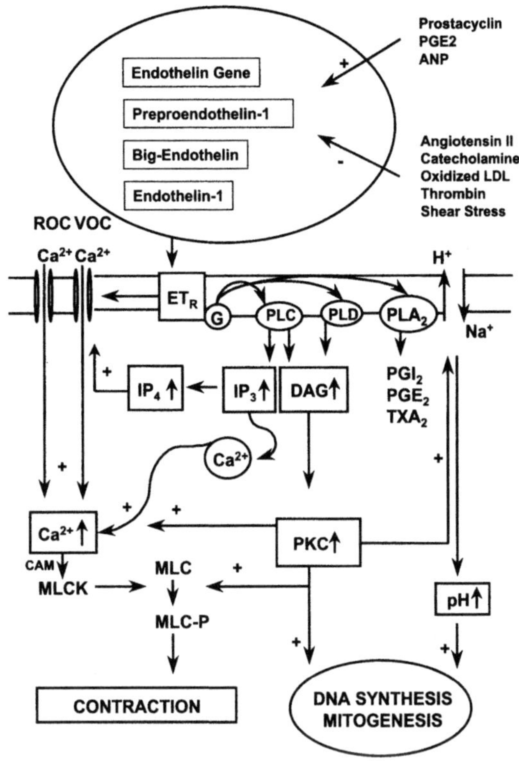

Fig. 4. Endothelin (ET) is a 22 amino acid peptide generated by proteolytic degradation from its precursor big-endothelin (big-ET). Various stimuli enhance others and inhibit the production of pre-pro-endothelin, the precursor of big-ET. The potent vasoconstrictor effects are mediated by activation of two distinct receptors ET_A and ET_B localized on smooth muscle cells and endothelial cells. Activation of the ET_A receptor predominately exerts the powerful vasoconstrictive effects at pharmacological and pathophysiological conditions by increasing intracellular Ca^{2+} levels. Signal transduction mechanisms involved in ET mediated long-term modulation of cell function (DNA synthesis, mitogenesis) include activation of proteinkinase C (PKC). PKC directly modulates cell function but also exerts indirect effects through elevation of intracellular pH (alkalization) via activation of Na^+/H^+ exchange. G, G-protein; PLC, PLD, $PLDA_2$, phospholipase C, D and A_2; IP_4, 1,3,4,5-inositol tetrakisphosphate; MLCK, myosin light chain kinase; DAG, diacylglycerol; ROC, receptor-operated calcium channel.

tion due to enhancement of intracellular calcium concentration. NO is known to shorten the duration of ET-1-mediated vasoconstriction most likely by accelerating the return of intracellular calcium to its basal concentration. Moreover, diacylglycerol and calcium stimulate protein kinase C, which mediates the long-term mitogenic action of ET-1 (Fig. 5).

Type B endothelin receptors are expressed predominantly on endothelial cells and to a much lesser extent on vascular smooth-muscle cells. ET-B receptors are linked to inhibitory G proteins, which in some cells leads to the inhibition of cyclic AMP generation and the activation of the Na^+/H^+ antiporter which may result in transient vasodilatation. The vasodilative properties of ET may also be caused at least in part by increased production of NO and prostacyclin and the activation of potassium channels.

Endothelin-1 is an important mediator of vascular tone in vivo and resembles a counterregulatory substance to NO under physiological conditions. Substances that enhance the production of ET-1 are angiotensin II, arginine vasopressin, thrombin, lipoproteins (HDL, LDL), and insulin. In addition, growth factors such as transforming growth factor β, insulin-like growth factor, epidermal growth factor, and basic fibroblast growth factors increase the concentration of bioactive ET-1. The stimulation of ET-1 production influences the effects of several other vasoactive substances and growth factors. In this regard it was demonstrated that ET-1 enhances the conversion of angiotensin-I to angiotensin-II and potentiated the angiotensin II-induced production of aldosterone (16).

The vasodilators NO and prostacyclin inhibit the production of ET-1 and its vasoconstrictive and mitogenic action. It might attenuate the increase of systemic vascular resistance that results from stimulation of ET-1 during high immunologic activity, hypoxia and increase in shear stress.

Signal transduction mechanisms of ET-1 involves short-term and long-term modulation of cell function. As outlined above, short-term effects of ET-1 include contraction of vascular smooth muscle by mobilization of intracellular Ca^{2+} and increased extracellular Ca^{2+} influx. Moreover, ET-1 potentiates the contractile response to other vasoconstrictor substances such as norepinephrine (NE) and serotonin. These findings implicate that ET-1-induced vasoconstriction is potentiated during disease states associated with inflammation.

In addition, ET-1 is known to activate phospholipase C (PLC) and D (PLD) in a receptor dependent manner (Fig. 3). This leads to activation of proteinkinase C (PKC) which results in activation of intranuclear *cfos* and *cjun*. It stimulates DNA synthesis and mitogenesis. Moreover, PKC stimulates the Na^+/H^+ antiporter which elevates intracellular pH and subsequently leads to increased DNA synthesis and mitogenesis resulting in smooth muscle cell migration and proliferation (16).

Recent evidence suggests that during myocardial ischemia and reperfusion the endogenous ET system is significantly activated. In addition, it has been demonstrated that supplementation of cardioplegia with a mixed ET-A/ET-B receptor antagonist and with the endothelin-converting enzyme inhibitor phosphoramidon improved post-ischemic myocardial function after prolonged hypothermic arrest. Importantly, there is evidence that, in conventional CPB, pulsatile flow conditions reduce endothelial cell activation as indicated by lower levels of cytokines and endothelin when compared to non-pulsatile flow. In addition, our own observations revealed that off-pump myocardial revascularization resulted in a significant reduction of the systemic big-endothelin levels when compared to conventional CPB, suggesting that extracorporeal circulation per se significantly contributes to endothelial cell activation (19).

Cardiopulmonary bypass and soluble cell adhesion molecules

The systemic inflammatory response during CPB contributes to increased cell adhesion due to expression of cell adhesion molecules. Despite early complement activation contributing to enhanced leukocyte adherence after CPB, which is short lived, a second more prolonged phase of increased cellular adhesion occurs in response to cytokines such as TNF-α or IL-6 which are activated proportionally to the duration of CPB. During this phase the activated endothelium undergoes profound alterations. Two important groups of cell adhesion molecules are the selectins (P- and E-selectin) and the immunoglobulin supergene family. The former are involved in the initial tethering and rolling process of activated leukocytes to the endothelial cell layer. P-selectin is stored in endothelial cells and is readily mobilized and released within minutes upon stimulation for example by TNF. E-selectin requires de novo synthesis and peaks within 4–6 hours after stimulation. For leukocytes to tether and role on the activated endothelium, they must express specific ligands. One important ligand for P-selectin is the P-selectin glycoprotein ligand (PSGL) which is expressed in lower concentration but exerts very high affinity for P-selectin expressed on the endothelial surface. PSGL-1 also interacts with E-selectin.

Despite the activation of the selectins, other important mediators involved in cell adhesion and transmigration are activated after CPB. One important adhesion molecule of the immunoglobulin supergene family is intracellular adhesion molecule 1 (ICAM-1). ICAM-1 is expressed constitutively in endothelial cells but up-regulation can be demonstrated after exposure to TNF. Induction of ICAM in response to cytokines requires translocation of at least two transcription factors NFκB and activator protein-1 (AP-1). ICAM-1 is critically involved in firm adhesion of leukocytes to endothelial cells. The importance of significant enhancement of tissue-specific adhesion molecules in myocardium and skeletal muscle after CPB has been demonstrated indicating that after the first wave of adherence is wearing off a second phase of increased cell adhesion molecule expression is present. It mediates a more prolonged leukocyte-endothelial interaction with the subsequent deleterious consequences. Because of the transient nature of endothelial cell activation following CPB most cells lose their increased state of adhesive properties shortly after the increased cytokine and complement (i.e., C5a) levels have returned to baseline values. In the majority of cardiac surgical procedures without any complications including infection or episodes of hypotension or shock, this appears within 24—72 h post surgery.

The role of the soluble forms of cell adhesion molecules which have been found to be increased under certain disease states such as after CPB remains uncertain. Encouraging results have been obtained from heart transplant recipients where elevated levels correlated with acute rejection episodes, thus permitting a differentiation between rejection episodes and stable graft function. However, others have shown that immunosuppressive drugs increase soluble adhesion molecule expression (3, 9).

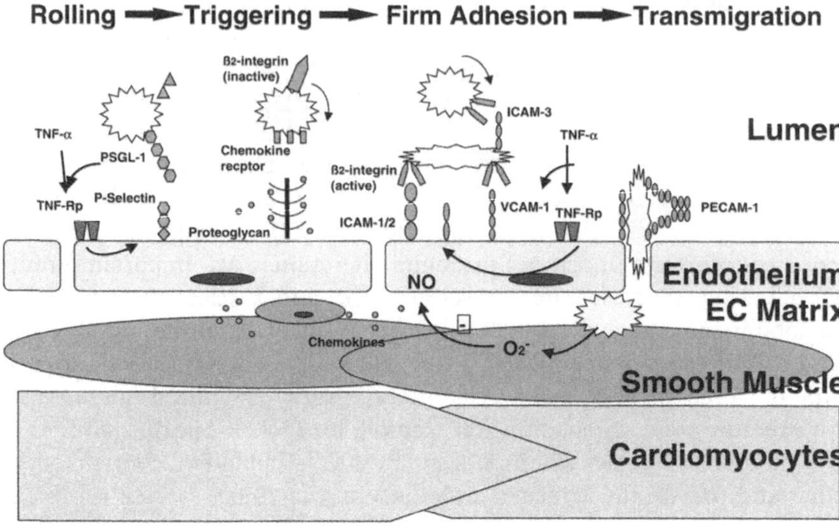

Fig. 5. Various steps leading to extravasation of inflammatory cells such as neutrophils are shown. During inflammation, leukocytes become activated thereby expressing P-selectin glycoprotein ligand-1 (PSFGL-1) which has high affinity for P-selectin on endothelial cells. Activated leukocytes become tethered to the luminal surface of the endothelium and subsequently roll along the endothelial surface as a consequence of the weak interaction between selectins and their ligands. At the inflammatory site, chemokines are released and become attached to proteoglycans on the endothelial surface where they are presented to rolling leukocytes. This results in intracellular signaling events with subsequent activation of the integrins. Upon integrin activation, leukocytes undergo conformational changes resulting in high-avidity binding with the immunoglobulin (Ig) supergene family endothelial ligands and firm adhesion of leukocytes to the endothelial surface. Once leukocytes have adhered firmly, they migrate towards endothelial cell junctions. PECAM-1 expression is concentrated on cellular junctions and mediates transmigration of leukocytes by engaging in homotypic interactions with leukocyte platelet – endothelial cell adhesion molecule (PECAM-1). Once the cells reached the interstitium, the leukocytes are thought to migrate through the extracellular matrix along a chemotactic gradient towards the inflammatory site.

Whether or not changes in levels of adhesion molecules following CPB simply reflect rather than mediate the inflammatory disease process remains elusive. However, soluble forms of adhesion molecules have been shown to be mediators of chronic inflammatory disease states such as in atherosclerosis. Our laboratory clearly demonstrated a significantly higher expression of P-selectin and ICAM-1 in conventional CABG patients when compared to those treated with OPCAB surgery. However, several study groups have demonstrated that levels of P-selectin decrease significantly or showed no alterations after CPB. The initial drop of P-selectin levels following CPB cannot be explained by hemodilution. However, since both platelet activation and platelet function are required for an increase in systemic P-selectin levels, it may be that either platelet activation does not occur during CPB or platelet function is significantly impaired.

Cardiopulmonary bypass and lipid peroxidation – evidence for oxyradical-mediated myocardial cell damage

Cardiopulmonary bypass exerts a disseminated intravascular postpump syndrome mediated by various factors such as the exposure of the organism to foreign surfaces, non-pulsatile flow conditions, and changes in shear stress conditions. Despite the systemic effects of CPB, the importance of oxyradical-mediated myocardial injury during CPB has been demonstrated in a variety of experimental and clinical settings. Most surgical procedures using CPB are associated with global myocardial ischemia induced by aortic cross clamping and subsequent reperfusion of the myocardium following aortic declamping; this results in considerable myocytolytic and microvascular damage, altered vasomotor function, and impaired vascular barrier function.

Important factors for myocardial injury during aortic cross clamping and CPB are a) the duration of myocardial ischemia and the duration of CPB, b) the temperature of the myocardium during ischemia, c) the method of myocardial preservation, and d) the quality of the reperfusate.

The duration of myocardial ischemia is reflected clinically by the development of myocardial stunning upon reperfusion. Stunning describes a reversible myocardial contractile dysfunction without morphological evidence for cellular injury and complete functional recovery within hours to days after initiation of reperfusion. In contrast to irreversibly injured hearts, the responsiveness of the stunned myocardium to catecholamines is adequate. Several mechanisms have been proposed to be responsible for stunning including formation of oxyradicals (superoxide, peroxynitrite), impaired availability of high energy phosphates, inhibition of Na^+/K^+-ATPase, inhibition of mitochondrial respiration, inactivation of sodium membrane channels, and activation of high output inducible nitric oxide synthase (iNOS) (15, 21).

The importance of temperature on the degree of cellular activation and release of pro-inflammatory mediators during CPB has been demonstrated. Moderate hypothermia (28–30 °C) has been shown to significantly reduce systemic cytokine release. In this regard, it has been reported that the temperature-dependent cytokine release was incriminated in the greater need for vasopressor support after normothermic CPB suggesting an enhanced cytokine-mediated vasoplegia in these patients (8).

A variety of cardioplegic solutions have been proposed to protect myocardial cellular integrity and function. Recent evidence suggests that blood cardioplegia reduces lipid peroxidation and troponin release during aortic unclamping. In addition, the need of electrical defibrillation was significantly higher in hearts preserved with crystalloid solutions when compared to cold blood cardioplegia.

Initiation of reperfusion following aortic declamping results in a burst of oxyradicals within the ischemic tissue. This is at least in part due to the increased formation of superoxide during ischemia subsequently leading to oxyradical formation upon reoxygenation. As a consequence, the release of highly reactive oxygen species leads to increased cellular alteration and injury. Indeed, several studies have demonstrated that cellular lipid peroxidation as demonstrated by increased malondialdehyde levels occurs after uncomplicated CPB. Moreover, recent evidence from our own observations demonstrates that myocardial and systemic lipid peroxidation products are significantly reduced in patients receiving off-pump CABG (OPCAB) surgery when comparing conventional CABG with CPB (Fig. 6). Recent reports suggest that the high iNOS/NO pathway significantly contribute to oxyradical damage by formation of peroxynitrite. It contributes to cellular damage, which may be detected by nitrotyrosine immunostaining. Our own laboratory has shown that selective modulation of the iNOS/NO pathway significantly reduces nitrotyrosine staining within myocardial microvascular endothelial cells. These findings suggest that strategies to prevent generation of radicals during CPB may improve postoperative morbidity and mortality (10, 11).

In addition to an enhanced cellular damage due to free radicals it has been demonstrated that myocardial injury as measured by creatinkinase or troponin levels is significantly greater in patients undergoing CPB when compared to PTCA or OPCAB procedures (Fig. 7). In the routine surgical patient this may not reflect a severe cardiac injury, since no significant hemodynamic impairment was observed in either group. However, in the critically ill patient or in patients with extended duration of CPB this may become a clinically relevant issue.

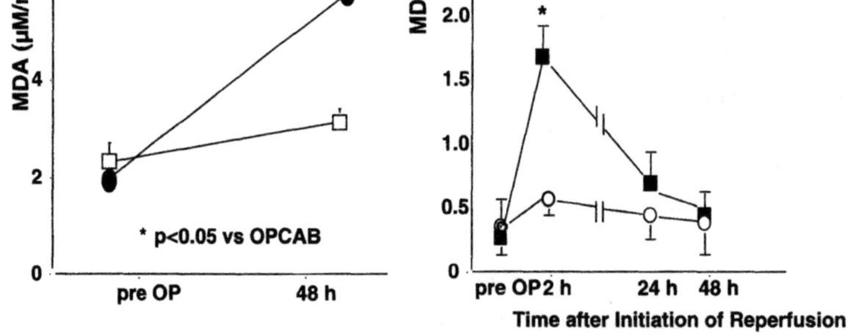

Fig. 6. A significant increase in plasma levels of malondialdehyde (MDA) was noted only in the patient group receiving conventional CABG using CPB (A). This was evident as early as 2 h after initiation of reperfusion. This was significantly different from the values measured in the OPCAB group. After 48 h of reperfusion MDA levels were found at baseline levels. *Indicates $P<0.05$ vs. pre-op levels; †indicates $P<0.05$ vs. OPCAB levels obtained at the same time interval.

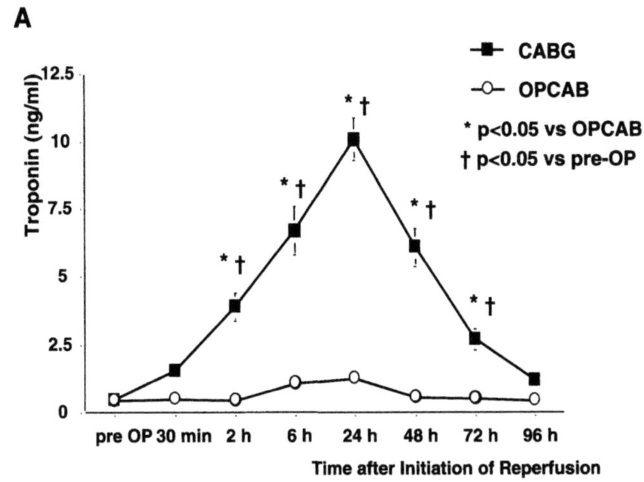

Fig. 7. Comparison of absolute values for troponin I (A) and creatinkinase MB fraction (CK-MB; B) between conventional (CABG) and off-pump CABG (OPCAB). Significant lower levels were observed over time in the OPCAB group (n=15) versus the CABG group (n = 17). Data were obtained in the absence of acute myocardial infarction or ischemia. *Indicates $P < 0.05$ vs. pre-op; †indicates $p < 0.05$ vs. OPCAB.

Therapeutic strategies

Hemodynamic instability and generalized organ dysfunction are common after CPB. As outlined in this review, several factors are involved in the alteration of vasomotor function and myocardial performance. Therapeutic options during CPB include the reduction of the systemic inflammatory response and lowering lipid peroxidation and myocardial cell damage.

The preservation of the vasodilatory state of the microvasculature is of major importance for regulation and adaptation of organ blood flow. Its improvement results in better organ function subsequently reducing morbidity and mortality. The clinical use of selective blockade of the endothelin system may be one strategy to improve organ perfusion. However, its value in routine cases remains to be established but it has been shown that non-specific ET receptor blockade by bosentan and BQ-123 improved low coronary flow during cardioplegic arrest. In addition, providing low concentrations of bioactive nitric oxide maintains a physiologic vasodilatory state and reduces cellular adhesion and inflammation. One primary therapeutic goal is therefore the enhanced protection of the endothelium and myocardium during ischemia. In this regard, various pharmacological approaches using antioxidants such as SOD, glutathione, and desferoxamine have been shown to significantly improve post-ischemic myocardial performance when given before the ischemic phase. In addition, exogenous NO donors such as sodium nitroprusside have been shown to be beneficial by alleviating the systemic and cardiac inflammatory response. Others have demonstrated that reduction of oxygen tension to normoxic conditions during reperfusion reduces the sources for oxyradical formation. Finally there is experimental and clinical evidence for novel and effective anti TNF-α strategies to be protective during CPB. For several years steroid administration and non-selective protease inhibitors have been used to reduce cytokine activation. Their benefit has been demonstrated by reduction in postoperative bleeding, improvement of lung function, and improvement of vascular barrier function. Recent data suggest that neutralization of TNF-α during sepsis by administration of soluble TNF receptors is safe and effective. Since TNF-α acts predominately in a paracrine fashion, its binding post-production may disarm the pro-inflammatory reaction. In this regard, it has been shown that antimurine TNF-α antibody improved postischemic left ventricular dysfunction.

Another anti-TNF strategy is the inhibition of the sphingomyelin metabolism by blocking the ceramidase enzyme (by N-oleoyl ethanolamine) within the sphingomyelin pathway; it has been shown to restore the TNF-induced contractile depression in cardiomyocyte culture.

In addition, several studies have demonstrated that selective iNOS inhibitors improve ventricular function by reduction of the high output NO pathway while preserving endothelial NO production. Selective iNOS inhibitors are S-methylisothiourea and several guanidine derivatives such as aminoguanidine or mercaptoethylguanidine.

Iron chelation by desferoxamine may protect against free radical formation. Despite its potent antioxidative effect, it also inhibits TNF-α production as has been shown to improve allograft survival after rat heterotopic cardiac transplantation.

The administration of anti-inflammatory cytokines such as IL-10 has been shown to inhibit TNF-α and reduced mortality during mice endotoxemia when given before the endotoxin challenge.

Several attempts have been made to reduce adhesion molecule expression on the endothelial surface. One non-specific but well established therapeutic and preventive approach is the use of protease inhibitors such as E-aminocapronic acid or aprotinin. It has been demonstrated that the administration of aprotinin prior to CPB significantly reduced P-selectin expression and the levels of conjugated dienes suggesting a reduction of endothelial activation and radical formation when compared to non-treated control patients. More selective ways to block cell adhesion include antibodies to P-selectin thereby reducing platelet adherence to endothelial cells. However, their usefulness in cardiac surgical procedures remains elusive.

References

1. Balligand J, Cannon P (1997) Nitric oxide synthases in cardiac muscle. Arteriosclerosis Thrombosis and Vascular Biology 17:1846–1858
2. Beyersdorf F, Mitrev Z, Sarai K, Eckel L, Klepzig H, Maul FD, Ihnken K, Satter P (1993) Changing patterns of patients undergoing emergency surgical revascularization for acute coronary occlusion. Importance of myocardial protection techniques. Journal of Thoracic and Cardiovascular Surgery 106:137–148
3. Boyle E, Pohlman T, Johnson M, Verrier E (1997) Endothelial cell injury in cardiovascular surgery: The systemic inflammatory response. Annals of Thoracic Surgery 63:277–284
4. Buckberg G (1995) Update on current techniques of myocardial protection. Annals of Thoracic Surgery 60:805–814
5. Cain B, Harken A, Meldrum D (1999) Therapeutic strategies to reduce TNF-α mediated cardiac contractile depression following ischemia and reperfusion. Journal of Molecular and Cellular Cardiology 31:931–947
6. DeMeules J, Pigula F, Mueller M, Raymond S, Gamelli R (1992) Tumor necrosis factor and cardiac function. Journal of Trauma 32:686–692
7. Drexler H (1999) Nitric oxide synthases in the failing human heart. Circulation 99:2972–2975
8. Ihnken K, Morita K, GD B, Sherman MP, Young HH (1995) Studies of hypoxemic/reoxygenation injury: Without aortic clamping. VI. Counteraction of oxidant damage by exogenous antioxidants: *N*-(2-mercaptopropionyl)-glycine and catalase. Journal of Thoracic and Cardiovascular Surgery 110(II):1212–1220
9. Jang Y, Lincoff A, Plow E, Topol E (1994) Cell adhesion molecules in coronary artery disease. Journal of American College of Cardiology 24:1591–1601
10. Liu P, Hock C, Nagele R, Wong P (1997) Formation of nitric oxide, superoxide, and peroxynitrite in myocardial ischemia-reperfusion injury in rats. American Journal of Physiology 272:H2327–H2336
11. Ma X, Lopez B, Liu G, Christopher T, Ischiropoulos H (1997) Peroxynitrite aggravates myocardial reperfusion injury in the isolated perfused rat heart. Cardiovascular Research 36:195–204
12. Moncada S, Palmer R, Higgs E (1991) Nitric oxide: physiology, pathophysiology, pharmacology. Pharmacological Reviews 43:109–142
13. Oral H, Dorn G, Mann D (1997) Sphingosine mediates the immediate negative inotropic effects of tumor necrosis factor-α in the adult mammalian cardiac myocyte. Journal of Biological Chemistry 272:4836–4842
14. Pilz G, Fraunberger P, Appel R, Kreuzer E, Werdan K, Walli A, Seidel D (1996) Early prediction of outcome in score-identified, postcardiac surgical patients at high risk for sepsis, using soluble tumor necrosis factor receptor-p55 concentrations. Critical Care Medicine 24:596–600
15. Piper H, Garcia-Dorado D, Ovize M (1998) A fresh look at reperfusion injury. Cardiovascular Research 38:291–300
16. Rubanyi G, Polokoff M (1994) Endothelins molecular biology, biochemistry, pharmacology, physiology, and pathophysiology. Pharmacological Reviews 46:325–415
17. Schulz R, Wambolt R (1995) Inhibition of nitric oxide synthesis protects the isolated working rabbit heart from ischemia-reperfusion injury. Cardiovascular Research 30:432–439
18. Wildhirt S, Schulze C, Conrad N, Kornberg A, Horstman D, Reichart B (1999) Aminoguanidine inhibits inducible NOS and reverses cardiac dysfunction late after ischemia and Reperfusion – Implications for iNOS mediated myocardial stunning. Thoracic- and Cardiovascular Surgeon 47:137–143
19. Wildhirt SM, Schulze C, Reichenspurner H, Conrad N, Rieder G, Boehm DH, Sreejayan N, Ritter C von, Welz A, Reichart B (1998) Gene expression of vasoactive mediators, myocardial lipidperoxidation and marker of cardiomyocyte damage after minimally invasive

(MIDCAB), port-access, and conventional cardiac operations. Thorac Cardiovasc Surg 46:189–190

20. Wildhirt S, Suzuki H, Horstman D, Weismueller S, Dudek R, Akiyama K, Reichart B (1997) Selective modulation of inducible nitric oxide synthase in myocardial infarction. Circulation 96:1616–1623
21. Wildhirt S, Weismueller S, Schulze C, Conrad N, Kornberg A, Reichart B (1999) Inducible nitric oxide synthase activation after ischemia and reperfusion contributes to myocardial dysfunction and extent of infarct size – evidence for a late phase of nitric oxide mediated reperfusion injury. Cardiovascular Research 43:698–711

Author's address:
Dr. Stephen M. Wildhirt
Herzchirurgische Klinik
Ludwig-Maximilians-Universität
Marchioninistr. 15
D-81377 München, Germany
e-mail: wildhirt@hch.med.uni-muenchen-de

Cytokine release regarding different perfusion systems and its effect on S100B protein levels

J. Babin-Ebell, M. Misoph, and O. Elert
Department of Cardiothoracic Surgery, University Hospital, Würzburg

Introduction

During cardiopulmonary bypass (CPB), blood is exposed to foreign surfaces and abnormal sheer forces. These abnormal conditions lead to an activation of coagulation (9), fibrinolysis (9), the complement pathway (2) and of the cellular and humoral immune system (15), finally resulting in a general inflammatory reaction. Clinically, this so-called "post pump response" is linked to myocardial dysfunction, respiratory distress, renal failure, and neurological deficits. All these clinical aspects are mostly consequences of endothelial injury and increased vascular permeability – at least partly caused by the release of cytokines, which are known to mediate vascular injury and organ dysfunction (4, 14).

In order to reduce the inflammatory response associated with CPB, the effects of oxygenator types, immunmodulation and heparin-coating have already been investigated. However, especially the effect of heparin-coating has been discussed controversially (8), and though an influence of abnormal sheer forces on complement activation and activation of leukocytes was pointed out already in the late 1980s (11), the effect of the conventional roller pump in comparison to the centrifugal pump on cytokine levels has not been investigated so far.

Additionally, it is of interest to investigate possible effects of this cytokine release.

Of all side effects of CPB, diffuse encephalopathy is a major and nearly regular cause of morbidity for patients undergoing CPB (16). Since the detection of these deficits depends on the timing of investigation and the test methods used, a simple laboratory marker indicating brain damage would make it much easier to quantify cerebral injury and to optimize the perfusion management and CPB set-up. The brain-specific isoenzyme of creatine phosphokinase failed to correlate with the occurrence of prolonged encephalopathy or stroke following CPB (3). Neuron-specific enolase (NSE) has been suggested as a marker for cerebral damage following CPB (1). However, the relevance of monitoring NSE may be limited by its presence in erythrocytes and platelets. Hemolysis due to the pump pressure and the artificial surfaces may thus reduce its specificity (13). S100 is an astroglial, calcium-binding protein, regulating cell growth, energy metabolism, and intracellular signal transduction. An elevation of its isoform S100B in cerebrospinal fluid and serum has already been linked to the extent of brain infarct, brain concussion, subarachnoidal hemorrhage, and encephalitis (20). Recently, the potential role of S100B as a marker for brain damage has been investigated in cardiac surgery (21).

Two principal reasons are discussed for neuropsychological deficits after CPB: multiple cerebral emboli (18) or an inflammatory reaction induced during CPB (10). To find responsible mechanisms for the S100B release and thus, hopefully, for cerebral dysfunction following CPB, we investigated whether S100B release can be correlated to embolus formation and/or to the release of inflammatory parameters.

Materials and methods

In all of our studies (only CABG patients), patients received a standard systemic heparin dose of 450 IU/kg and a low dose aprotinin regimen (2×10^6 units at skin incision and 500000 units/h until the end of the operation). The ACT was kept above 450 s. For comparative investigations on biocompatibility, either a Medtronic Biomedicus centrifugal pump, a Stöckert roller pump or a Medtronic Biomedicus centrifugal pump combined with Carmeda heparin-coated surfaces was used. Pump flow was non-pulsatile and corresponded to 2.5 $l/min/m^2$ body surface as 100% cardiac output. The operation was performed in moderate hypothermia with a rectal temperature between 30 and 32 °C.

The concentrations of interleukin 6 and –8 and of C5a were determined by ELISA, that of S100B by the Byk-Sangtec LIA. Release of these parameters was calculated by integrating the relevant curves (area under curve).

For embolus detection (high intensity transient signals, HITS), a Hatteland microbubble ultrasound detector was used at the arterial line of CPB.

Results and discussion

Of all cytokines both IL-6 and IL-8 have been most tightly linked to patients outcome (4, 14). Several studies have confirmed that IL-6 regulates the synthesis of acute phase proteins and is most likely a major regulator of the acute phase reaction. Furthermore, IL-6 has negative inotropic effects, occurring within minutes after administration. The level of IL-6 production has been correlated to the duration of non-CPB operations (6) and may be a marker of tissue injury of the operation itself (19). However, besides operation trauma, CPB itself leads to an elevation of IL-6 levels, which has clearly been demonstrated by CPB-supported PTCA (17). In our investigation, IL-6

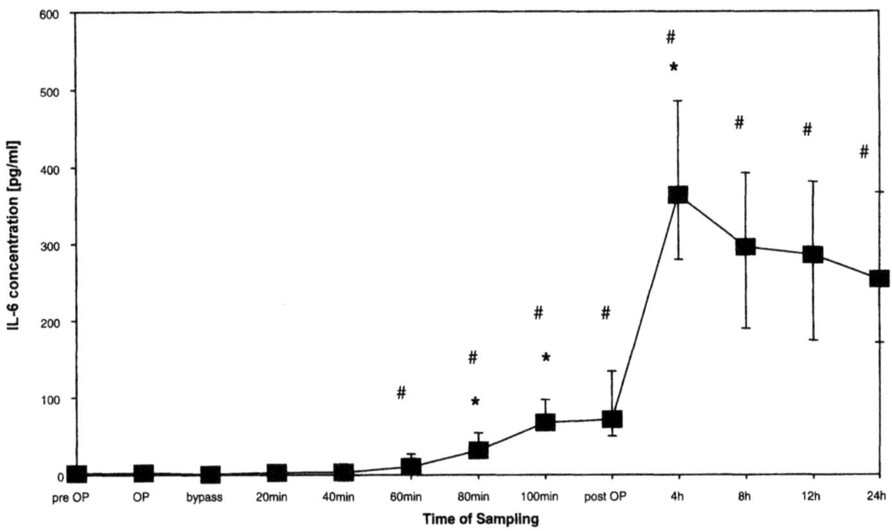

Fig. 1. Interleukin 6 plasma concentration of 27 patients undergoing CABG with CPB and a centrifugal pump. Data are presented as medians with lower and upper quartiles. *: Value significantly different to preceeding value; #: value significantly different to pre OP value ($p \leq 0.05$; Wilcoxon signed rank test). Sampling time points: pre OP: 2–3 h prior to surgery; OP: right before the onset of CPB; bypass: immediately after the onset of CPB; 20–100 min: every 20 min during CPB; post OP: after protamine administration; 4 h, 8 h, 12 h, 24 h postoperatively.

levels increased in the late phase of CPB and remained highly elevated further on (Fig. 1).

IL-8 is secreted by macrophages and endothelial cells. It induces leukocyte adherence to vascular endothelium and their extravasation into tissues. It is suggested that IL-8 is responsible for neutrophil activation and cell injury (14). Its release may play a role in the pathophysiology of capillary leak through neutrophil degranulation (7) and seems to be involved in multi-organ failure (4). In the plasma of our patients, IL-8 concentrations (Fig. 2) reached their maximum postoperatively and returned to normal in the following 24 h.

IL-10 is known as an antiinflammatory cytokine. It suppresses, for example, the release of TNF-α and IL-8. In our patients, IL-10 concentrations started to rise already after 60 minutes CPB duration (Fig. 3), possibly indicating the activation of an early anti-inflammatory response to CPB.

Several studies demonstrated a better blood handling by the centrifugal pump in comparison to the conventional roller pump. Hence, theoretically, by reduction of sheer stress application of the centrifugal pump could lead to reduced cytokine release. However, in our studies the release of IL-6, IL-8, and IL-10 during the investigated time period – calculated as area under curve – was not significantly different between the patient group receiving a roller pump and that with a centrifugal pump (Table 1). We could thus not demonstrate a positive effect of the centrifugal pump on cytokine levels.

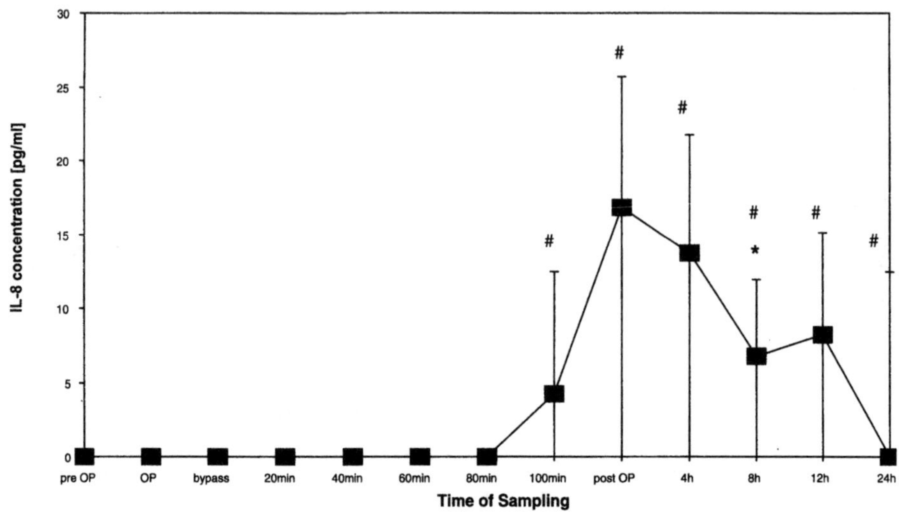

Fig. 2. Interleukin 8 plasma concentration of 27 patients undergoing CABG with CPB and a centrifugal pump. Data are presented as medians with lower and upper quartiles. *: Value significantly different to preceeding value; #: value significantly different to pre OP value ($p \leq 0.05$; Wilcoxon signed rank test). Sampling time points: pre OP: 2–3 h prior to surgery; OP: right before the onset of CPB; bypass: immediately after the onset of CPB; 20–100 min: every 20 min during CPB; post OP: after protamine administration; 4 h, 8 h, 12 h, 24 h postoperatively.

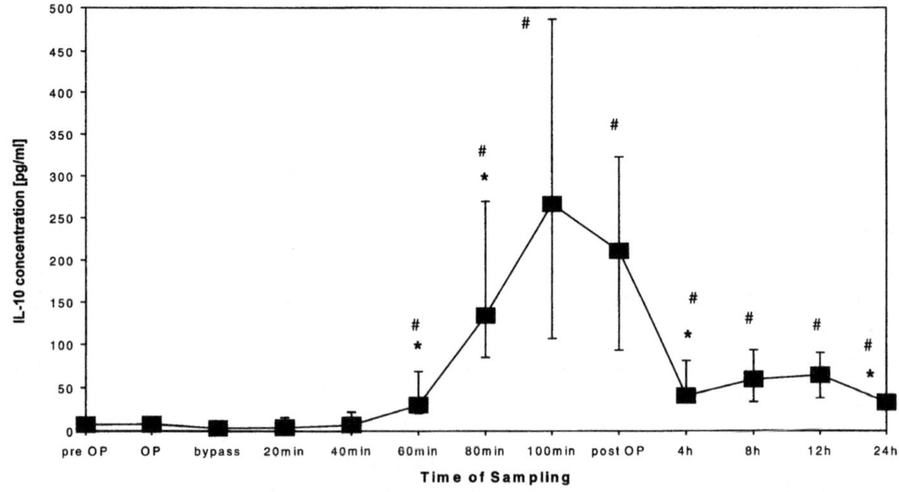

Fig. 3. Interleukin 10 plasma concentration of 27 patients undergoing CABG with CPB and a centrifugal pump. Data are presented as medians with lower and upper quartiles. *: Value significantly different to preceeding value; #: value significantly different to pre OP value ($p \leq 0.05$; Wilcoxon signed rank test). Sampling time points: pre OP: 2–3 h prior to surgery; OP: right before the onset of CPB; bypass: immediately after the onset of CPB; 20–100 min: every 20 min during CPB; post OP: after protamine administration; 4 h, 8 h, 12 h, 24 h postoperatively.

Table 1. Release of pro- and anti-inflammatory cytokines in patients undergoing CPB in dependence of the used pump system

Parameter	Group RP	Group CP	p-value
IL-6	1522 (1028–1915)	1140 (855–1655)	n. s.
IL-8	49 (19–75)	52 (23–103)	n. s.
IL-10	696 (372–1087)	614 (316–940)	n. s.

Data are presented as medians with lower and upper quartiles in parenthesis and calculated as areas under curve during investigation time. RP: roller pump group; CP: centrifugal pump group; n. s.: not significant, $p \leq 0.05$ (nonparametric U-test for unpaired samples of Wilcoxon, Mann and Whitney).

Table 2. Release of pro- and anti-inflammatory cytokines in patients undergoing CPB in dependence of the surface of the CPB system

Parameter	Group CP	Group CPhc	p-value
IL-6	1140 (855–1655)	1315 (740–1555)	n. s.
IL-8	52 (23–103)	31 (14–93)	n. s.
IL-10	614 (316–940)	647 (449–1548)	n. s.

Data are presented as medians with lower and upper quartiles in parenthesis and calculated as areas under curve during investigation time. CP: centrifugal pump group; CPhc: centrifugal pump group with heparin-coated CPB surfaces; n. s.: not significant, $p \leq 0.05$ (nonparametric U-test for unpaired samples of Wilcoxon, Mann and Whitney).

Though the beneficial effect of heparin-coated surfaces is discussed controversially, a reduction of complement activation has been demonstrated in several investigations (12). Since complement-derived fragments may increase production of IL-1, TNF-α and IL-6 (5), a reduction of cytokine release during and after CPB by heparin-coating could be assumed. In contrast, in our studies the release of IL-6, IL-8, and IL-10 during the investigated time period – again calculated as area under curve – was not significantly different between the patient group receiving heparin-coated surfaces and that with an uncoated CPB system (Table 2). Thus, we could not demonstrate a positive effect of a heparin-coated CPB system on cytokine levels.

Multiple cerebral emboli (18) and/or the inflammatory reaction induced during CPB (10) are discussed as reasons for the neuropsychological deficits after CPB. Hence it was of interest to investigate whether S100B-release can be correlated to embolus formation and/or to the release of inflammatory parameters to be thus able to distinguish between the possible mechanisms for the S100B-release and thus for cerebral dysfunction following CPB.

Confirming the results of other studies, in our patients we could also observe an elevation of S100B concentration during CPB (Fig. 4).

To obtain a standardized time course for embolus detection in each patient, embolus count was performed for 3 min after start of CPB, for 10 min after cross-clamping, 10 min after the beginning of rewarming, and 10 min

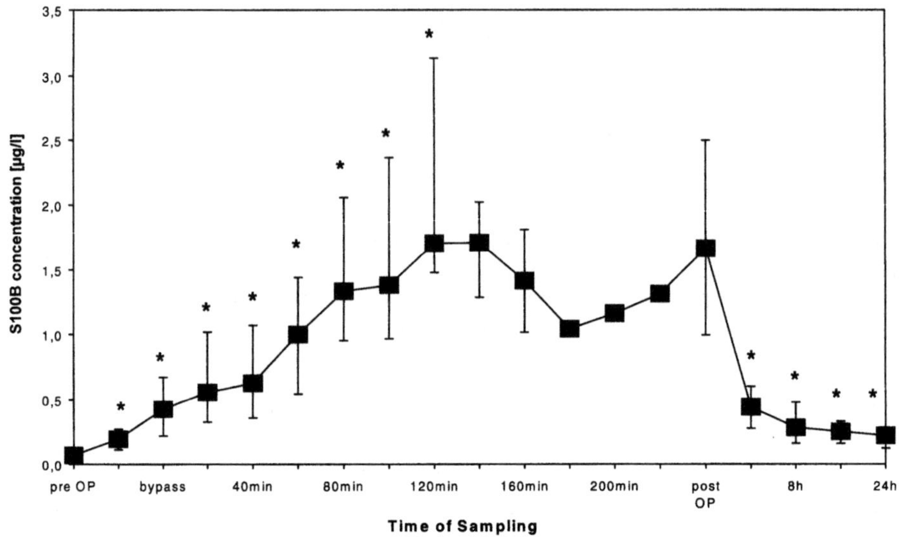

Fig. 4. S100B concentration in 40 patients undergoing CABG with CPB. Data are presented as medians with lower and upper quartiles. *: Value significantly different to preceeding value (p ≤0.05; Wilcoxon signed rank test). Sampling time points: pre OP: 2–3 h prior to surgery; OP: right before the onset of CPB; bypass: immediately after the onset of CPB; 20–220 min: every 20 min during CPB; post OP: after protamine administration; 4 h, 8 h, 12 h, 24 h postoperatively.

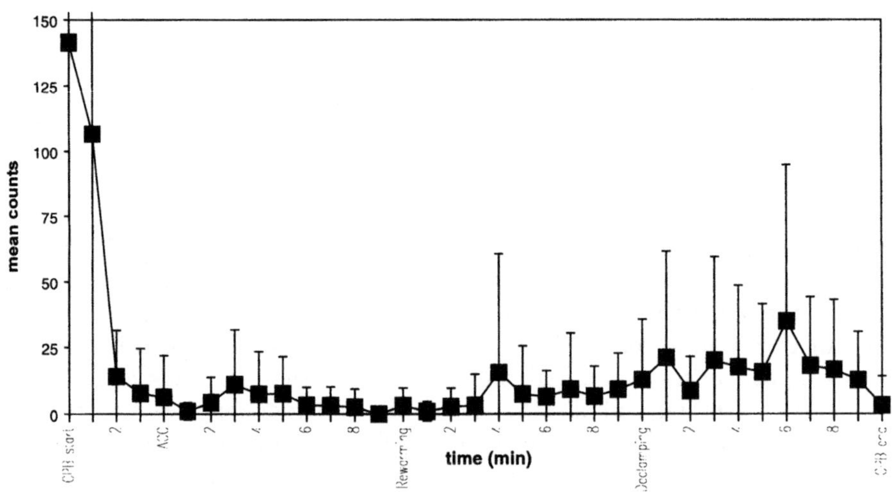

Fig. 5. Embolus count at standardized time intervals in patients undergoing CABG with CPB. Data are presented as means with standard deviation.

after declamping. Embolus detection at the arterial line of 20 patients (Fig. 5) revealed a peak at the onset of CPB, only few counts during the initial phase of CPB and a moderate increase in microbubble formation during rewarming.

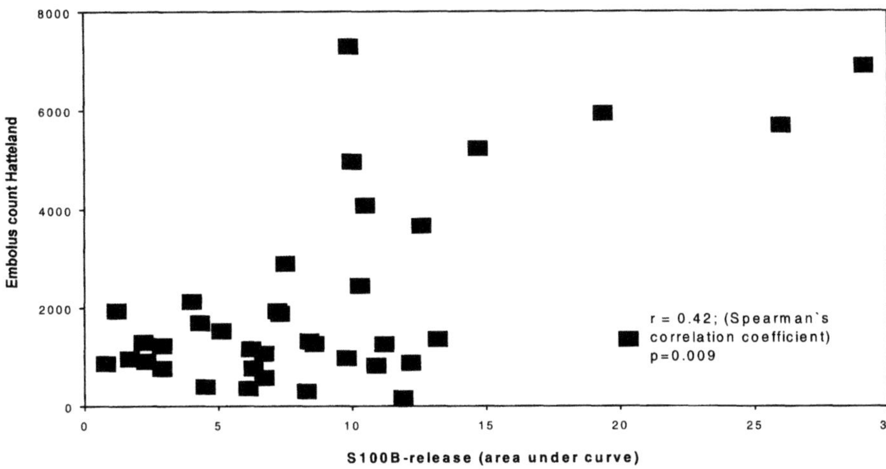

Fig. 6. Correlation of S100B-release and embolus count in 40 patients undergoing CABG with CPB.

Table 3. Correlation of S100B-release with embolus count and inflammatory parameters

Parameter	r_s	p-value	r_p	p-value
Embolus count	0.42	0.009	0.57	<0.0001
IL-8-release	0.58	<0.0001	0.29	n. s.
C5a-formation	–0.02	n. s.	–0.14	n. s.

r_s: Spearman's correlation coefficient; r_p: partial correlation coefficient; n. s.: not significant, $p \leq 0.05$ (nonparametric U-test for unpaired samples of Wilcoxon, Mann and Whitney).

To investigate whether there is a correlation between the number of intraoperative emboli and S100B-release, the area under the S100B curve was calculated as a measure for the S100B-release and plotted against the total embolus count (number of all emboli during CPB). We found a significant correlation of both parameters (Fig. 6), indicating that the release of S100B could be due to intraoperative embolus formation.

Regarding the effect of inflammatory parameters on the S100B-release, we could not find a correlation of S100B-release and C5a-formation. Moreover, the correlation of S100B- and IL-8-release was found to be due to a third parameter affecting both of them, namely, CPB time. Hence, when a partial correlation was performed with CPB time as the control variable, the correlation of S100B and IL-8 vanished (Table 3).

Conclusions

We could demonstrate an inflammatory reaction of CABG with CPB. However, the investigated perfusion systems – Medtronic Biomedicus centrifugal pump and Carmeda heparin-coating – did not affect cytokine release differently when compared to the conventional system.

Embolus detection revealed a peak in embolus formation at the onset of CPB, only few counts during the initial phase of operation and again an increase during rewarming. These emboli seem to cause a S100B-release. In contrast, inflammatory parameters (IL-8 and C5a) were not found to be responsible for cerebral damage during CPB.

References

1. Aberg T (1995) Signs of brain cell injury during open heart operations: past and present. Ann Thorac Surg 59:1312–1315
2. Bonser RS, Dave J, Gademsetty M, Carter P, Davies E, Taylor P, Gaya H, Lennox SC, Vergani D (1990) Complement activation before, during and after cardiopulmonary bypass. Eur J Cardio-thorac Surg 4:291–296
3. Breuer AC, Furlan AJ, Hanson MR et al (1983) Central nervous system complications of coronary artery bypass graft surgery: prospective analysis of 421 patients. Stroke 14:682–687
4. Casey LC (1993) Role of cytokines in the pathogenesis of cardiopulmonary-induced multisystem organ failure. Ann Thorac Surg 56:92–96
5. Cavaillon JM, Fitting C, Haeffner-Cavaillon N (1990) Recombinated C5a enhances interleukin 1 and tumor necrosis factor release by lipopolysaccharid-stimulated monocytes and macrophages. Eur J Immunol 20:253–257
6. Cruickshank AM, Fraser WD, Burns HJ, Van Damme J, Shenkin A (1990) Response of serum interleukin-6 in patients undergoing elective surgery of varying severity. Clin Sci Colch 79:161–165
7. Finn A, Naik S, Klein N, Levinsky R, Strobel S, Elliott M (1993) Interleukin-8 release and neutrophil degranulation after pediatric cardiopulmonary bypass. J Thorac Cardiovasc Surg 105:234–241
8. Gorman RC, Ziats NP, Rao AK, Gikakis N, Sun L, Kahn MMH, Stenach N, Sapatnekar S, Chouhan V, Gorman JH, Niewiarowski S, Colman RW, Anderson JM, Edmunds LH (1996) Surface-bound heparin fails to reduce thrombin formation during clinical cardiopulmonary bypass. J Thorac Cardiovasc Surg 111:1–12
9. Grossmann R, Babin-Ebell J, Misoph M, Schwender S, Neukam K, Hickethier Th, Elert O, Keller F (1996) Changes in coagulation and fibrinolytic parameters caused by extracorporeal circulation. Heart Vessels 11:310–317
10. Hennein HA, Ebba H, Rodriguez JL, Merrick SH, Keith FM, Bronstein MH, Leung JM, Mangano DT, Greenfield LJ, Rankin JS (1994) Relationship of the proinflammatory cytokines to myocardial ischemia and dysfunction after uncomplicated coronary revascularization. J Thorac Cardiovasc Surg 108:626–635
11. Jakob H, Kutschera Y, Palzer B, Prellwitz W, Oelert H (1990) In-Vitro Assessment of Centrifugal Pumps for Ventricular Assist. Artif Organs 14(4):278–283
12. Jansen PGM, te Velthuis H, Huybregts RAJM, Paulus R, Bulder ER, van der Spoel HI, Bezemer PD, Slaats EH, Eijsman L, Wildevuur CHR (1995) Reduced complement activation and improved postoperative performance after cardiopulmonary bypass with heparin-coated circuits. J Thorac Cardiovasc Surg 110:829–834
13. Johnsson P (1996) Markers of cerebral ischemia after cardiac surgery. J Cardiothorac Vasc Anesth 10:120–126
14. Kawamura T, Wakusawa R, Kazutoshi O, Inada S (1993) Elevation of cytokines during open heart surgery with cardiopulmonary bypass: participation of interleukin 8 and 6 in reperfusion injury. Can J Anaesth 40(11):1016–1021

15. Misoph M, Babin-Ebell J (1997) Interindividual variations in cytokine levels following cardiopulmonary bypass. Heart Vessels 12:119–127
16. Murkin JM (1995) The role of CPB management in neurobehavioural outcomes after cardiac surgery. Ann Thorac Surg 59:1308–1311
17. Prodzinsky R, Witthaut R, Stabenow I, Lehrmann D, Redling F, Fraunberger P, Walli AK, Seidel D, Zerkowski HR, Teichmann W, Werdan K (1997) The cardiopulmonary bypass supported high-risk PTCA (CPB-PTCA): a useful model for the study of CPB-dependent systemic inflammatory response syndrom (SIRS)? Crit Care 1(Suppl 1):S41
18. Pugsley W, Klinger L, Paschalis C, Treasure T, Harrison M, Newman S (1994) The impact of microemboli during cardiopulmonary bypass on neuropsychological functioning. Stroke 25:1393–1399
19. Shenkin A, Fraser WD, Series J, Winstanley FP, McCartney AC, Burns HJ, Van Damme J (1989) The serum interleukin 6 response to elective surgery. Lymphokine Res 8:123–127
20. Waterloo K, Ingebritsen T, Romner B (1997) Neuropsychological function in patients with increased serum levels of protein S-100 after minor head injury. Acta Neurochir Wien 139:26–32
21. Westaby S, Johnsson P, Parry AJ et al (1996) Serum S100 protein: a potential marker for cerebral events during cardiopulmonary bypass. Ann Thorac Surg 61:88–92

Author's address:
Dr. Jörg Babin-Ebell
Klinik und Poliklinik für Herz- und Thoraxchirurgie
Universität Würzburg
Josef-Schneider-Str. 6
D-97080 Würzburg, Germany

$SMAR_xT$ and blood air interface – a new concept to improve biocompatibility of extracorporeal circuits –

F. Isgro, A.-H. Kiessling, and W. Saggau
Department of Cardiac Surgery, Heart Center Ludwigshafen, Germany

Introduction

Cardiopulmonary bypass (CPB) alters the immunologic host response by activation of both, the humoral and the cellular components of the immune system. During CPB, artificial surfaces and filters coated with plastics, glass or metal, and the cardiotomy suction, aspiration, and blood air interface result in many alterations in structure and function of the blood that passes through the extracorporeal circuit and indirectly into the tissues.

When blood first contacts the foreign materials of the circuit, platelets adhere to the surface and Hageman factor activation and subsequently activation of kallikrein, the kinin-bradykinin system, and the fibrinolytic and complement cascade are initiated. Platelets undergo morphologic changes consistent with activation during CPB, releasing β-thromboglobulin (β-TG) into the plasma. Protein S100B and neuronspecific enolase (NSE) as biochemical markers of cerebral injury and increased permeability of the blood brain barrier leak into the blood during CPB and are predictors of central nervous system complications.

The purpose of our study was to compare the effects of $SMAR_xT$ circuits in combination with a modified aspiration management on platelet and cerebral markers including a neuropsychometric test (MMST) and also on various markers of the inflammatory response.

Materials and methods

The study was perfomed as a prospective, randomized, double-blind clinical trial, comprising 80 patients between the ages of 18 and 75 with a body weight greater than 60 kilograms, who were scheduled for elective coronary artery bypass graft operations. The patients were randomly divided into two subgroups.

In one subgroup $SMAR_xT$ circuit components were used. In the other, standard untreated circuits were used.

Exclusion criteria were as follows:
- psychiatric or neurologic illness

- severe dysfunction of the kidney and liver
- severe dysfunction of the hematopoetic system
- diagnosed cancer
- emergency operation
- re-operation

The oxygenators used in this study were flat sheet membrane oxygenators manufactured by Cobe Cardiovascular, Inc. For the standard circuits, the oxygenator was the standalone CML DUO™ Disposable Blood Oxygenator. For the "biocompatible" circuit the oxygenator was the CML DUO™ Disposable Blood Oxygenator with SMA. Both membrane compartments had been used for all patients. The arterial filter was the Cobe Sentry™ Arterial Filter with SMA for the SMAR$_x$T patients and the Cobe Sentry™ with Primegard for the control. The venous blood reservoir was the COBE VRB-1800, one with SMA and one without.

The aspiration management was optimized as follows:
- totally closed system
- no coronary suction
- modified vent
- cell saver
- no shed blood retransfused

Venous blood samples were collected on 7 occasions:
- T1: preoperative
- T2: ECC –5 min
- T3: ECC +20 min
- T4: cross-clamp +5 min
- T5: protamine +10 min
- T6: postoperative +4 h
- T7: postoperative +24 h

On each sample, plasma β-TG levels, concentrations of protein S100B and NSE were measured. Additionally, routine hematological markers as well as markers of the inflammatory response were determined. The Mini-Mental Status Test (MMST) as neuropsychological screening was performed preoperatively and 5 days postoperatively.

Results

Demographics (Tables 1 and 2)

There were no significant differences between the groups with regard to age, body mass index, sex, CPB time, cross-clamp time, and operation duration. Two dropouts had to be substituted due to surgical complications.

Table 1. Patient characteristics

	SMAR$_x$T group	Control group
Patients	n = 40	n = 40
Sex	35 male	32 male
Age	64 yrs	65.2 yrs
Body mass index	1.9 m^2	2.0 m^2

Table 2. Operation averages

Duration	SMAR$_x$T group	Control group
Operation time	173.2 min (n.s.)	165.9 min (n.s.)
Bypass time	67.9 min (n.s.)	70.6 min (n.s.)
Cross clamping time	40.8 min (n.s.)	41.8 min (n.s.)

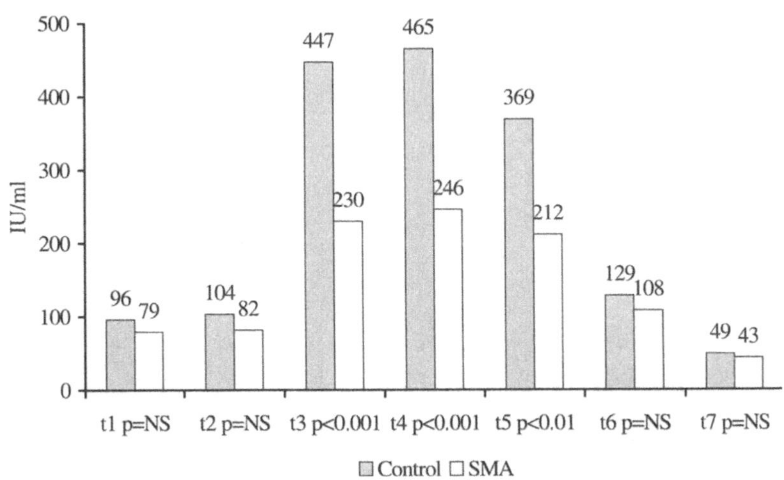

Fig. 1. Mean values of β-thromboglobulin. Plasma levels of β-thromboglobulin increased significantly in both groups 20 min after the beginning of CPB (T3) with peak levels 5 min after the release of the cross-clamp (T4). Four hours postoperatively (T6) the levels decreased toward preoperative levels (T1). A significant difference between SMAR$_x$T and control patients was registered at T3, T4, and T5 ($p \leq 0.001$ (T3+T4); $p \leq 0.01$ (T5)) being lower in the SMAR$_x$T group.

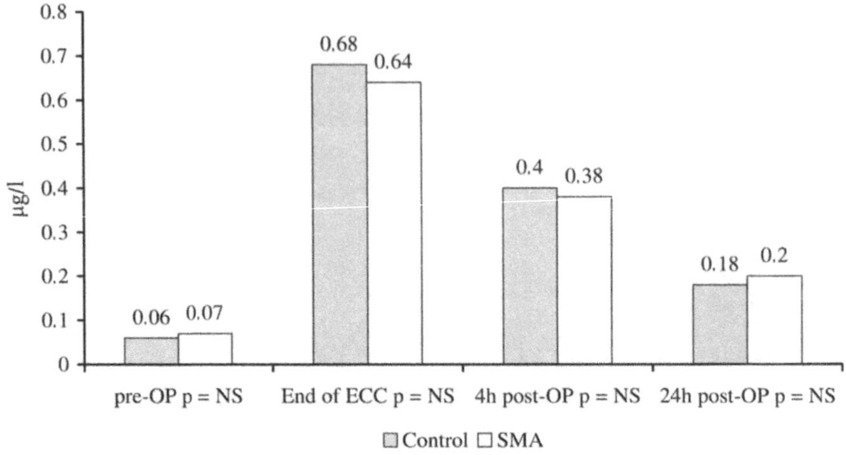

Fig. 2. Mean values of S100B protein. Protein S100B plasma concentrations peaked in both groups after termination of CPB (T5) reaching levels of 0.64+0.33 µg/l (SMAR$_x$T) and 0.68+0.42 µg/l (control) compared to preoperative levels of 0.06+0.06 µg/l for both groups. Four hours postoperatively (T6) a recovery of the protein S100B concentrations was observed (0.38+0.24 µg/l (SMAR$_x$T); 0.41+0.27 µg/l (control)), while 24 hours postoperatively S100B levels returned almost to the preoperative levels in both groups. The difference between the two groups did not reach statistical significance at any time.

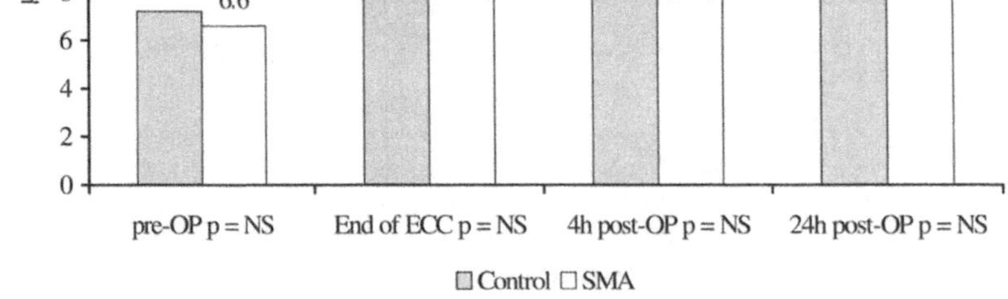

Fig. 3. Mean values of neuronspecific enolase (NSE). Plasma concentrations of neuronspecific enolase (NSE) increased continously during the operation reaching a maximum 24 hours postoperatively (T7) (15.7+6.2 µmol/l (SMAR$_x$T) vs. 16.2+8.3 µmol/l (control)). Although the NSE levels at all sampling times were higher in the control group, the difference did not reach statistical significance.

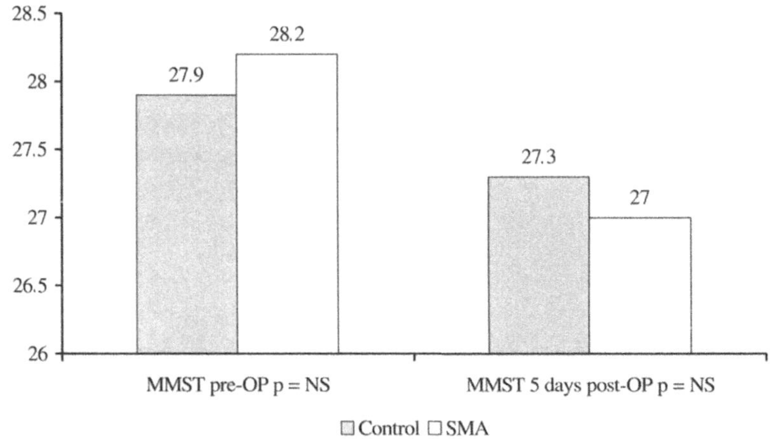

Fig. 4. Mean values of Mini-Mental Status Test (MMST). The Mini-Mental Status Test was performed preoperatively and on postoperative day 5. A point loss of 3 or more was considered as pathological. Preoperative test results were equal in both groups (28.2±1.4 points (SMAR$_x$T) vs 27.9±1.9 points (control)). Also the mean values 5 days postoperative were not significantly different (27.0±4.9 p (SMAR$_x$T) vs 27.3±2.7 p (control)). Nevertheless, in 8 patients a point loss of 3 or more could be registered and 6 of them belonged to the control group and only 2 received SMARxT circuits.

Discussion

In the present trial, the use and usefulness of extracorporeal circuits treated with surface modifying additives (SMA) has to asked critically. But it is not only surface modification that is a major source of blood activation, but more so the modification of the blood air interface. It is well documented that aspirated blood is highly activated and furthermore the air blood mixture will cause platelet and leucocyte activation promoting the release of vasoactive and toxic substances. Thus, we changed our protocol in order to minimize this blood-air interaction.

This modification of the aspiration management (e.g., no coronary suction, cardiotomy blood treated with cell saver before retransfused, modified vent) may be the explanation for the remarkably low peak levels of protein S100 and NSE compared to other studies, focusing on the pathophysiology of CPB. But it seems to be not only a biochemical gambling with cerebral ischemia markers but rather an improvement of neuropsychological outcome as shown by the results of the Mini-Mental Status Test.

Without doubt the most striking effect of SMAR$_x$T treated circuits is on platelet function. Platelet preservation is much better in patients with SMAR$_x$T circuits as revealed by considerably lower peak levels of β-thromboglobulin.

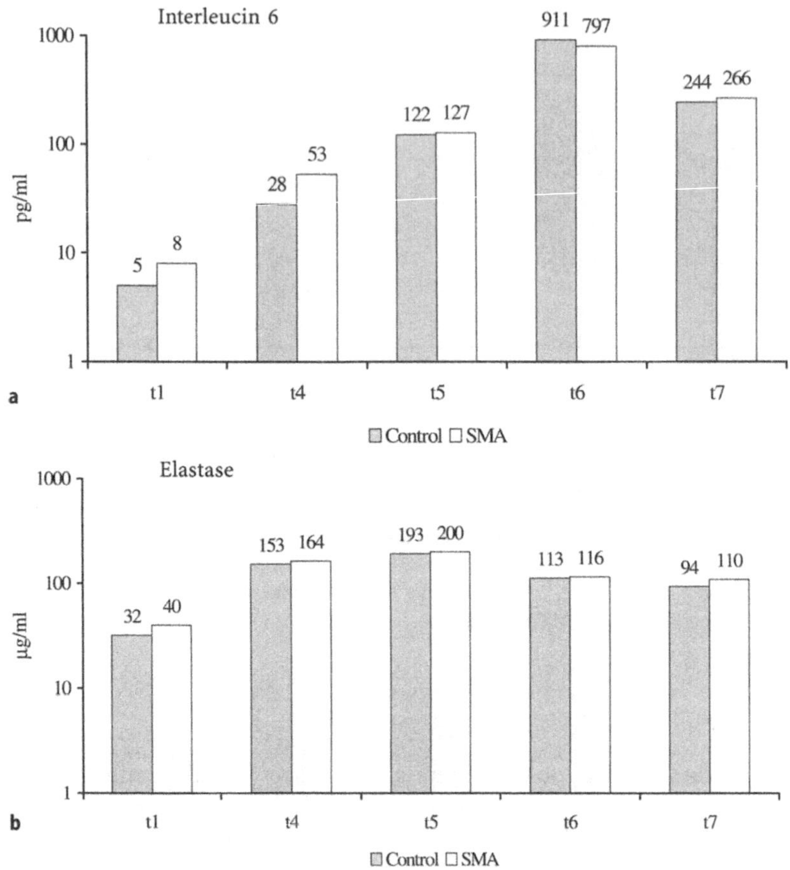

Fig. 5. (**a**) Mean values of interleukin 6; (**b**) Mean values of elastase. Both markers of inflammatory response increased during and after CPB showing the classical, well known kinetics. However, the difference between the two groups never reached statistical significance.

Conclusion

Despite the subordinate effects of SMAR$_x$T circuits on the inflammatory markers, the use of these circuits definitely preserves platelet function much better compared to standard circuits, with the potential to reduce blood loss and transfusion of blood products. In addition, a positive effect on cerebral outcome can be presumed, particularly in combination with an optimized blood air interface with a direct impact on the clinical outcome of the patients, which should be our main target.

Author's address:
Dr. Frank Isgro
Herzzentrum Ludwigshafen
Klinik für Herzchirurgie
Bremserstr. 79
D-67063 Ludwigshafen, Germany

Impact of the cardiopulmonary bypass circuit on brain dysfunction – detection of microemboli by transcranial Doppler ultrasound: preliminary comparative data on flat sheet vs. hollow fiber oxygenators

H.-R. Zerkowski, M. Preiss, M. Walenta, and F. Bernet
Clinic of Cardio-Thoracic Surgery, Kantonsspital Basel,
Universitätskliniken, Basel, Switzerland

Brain injury remains a significant problem in patients undergoing cardiac surgery using cardiopulmonary bypass (CPB) despite continuous improvements in surgical technique, anesthesia management, and CBP equipment (type of oxygenator, gradients in the heat exchanger, intracardiac sucker systems). Although the cause of brain injury during cardiac surgery is certainly multifactorial, evidence suggests that microemboli play an important role because embolized particles cause transient obstructions to flow (Fig. 1). Evidence linking microemboli to neurological complications is supported by studies using carotid and transcranial Doppler ultrasound (TCD) (6, 11, 18). The number of emboli correlates well with early neuropsychological deficits and risk of stroke as well as length of hospital stay (15). Incidence rates for stroke are around 2% to 3% (5) and may be contrasted with the much higher reported incidence of cognitive defects assessed by neuropsychological testing (1). There are a variety of ways, at least potentially, in which the brain may be injured during an operation with CPB, including reduced cerebral blood flow, microembolism, and systemic inflammatory response (Table 1). Cerebral microemboli are known to occur during specific surgical interventions, but the source of a large proportion of emboli remains unexplained. Also important is, that interventions of the perfusionist could account for the appearance of cerebral microemboli (16). Many sources of microemboli during open heart surgery have been suggested, including microembolism of air, fat, platelet aggregate or silicone (5, 13).

This study was undertaken to determine the influence of the membrane oxygenators of Cobe[1] (Cobe Lab., Lakewood, CO) or Dideco[2] (Dideco S.A. Mirandola, Italy) associated with their ability to eliminate microemboli measured as high intensity signals in Doppler ultrasound.

---

[1] Cobe CML DUO™
[2] Dideco D 703 Compactflo™

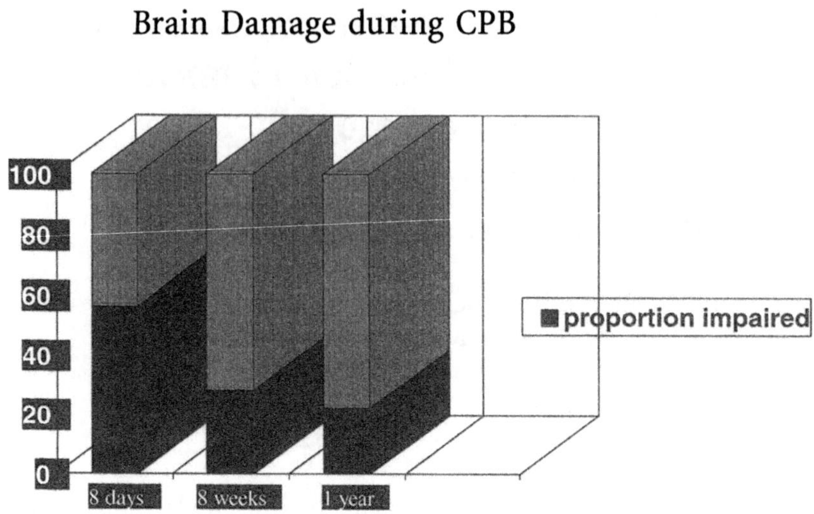

Fig. 1. Incidence of cognitive defects compared to preoperative level in patients undergoing coronary artery bypass grafting (Smith PLC (1998) Ann R Surg Engl 70:212–216).

Table 1. MES (microemboli signals) and cardiovascular disease; [ATS; SJM: trademarks of heart valves/DCM: dilatative cardiomyopathy]

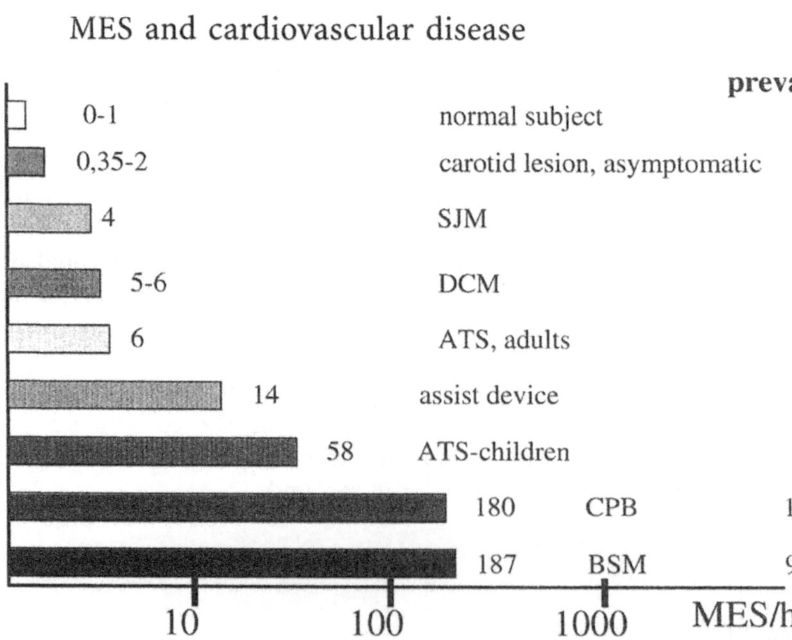

Brain injury due to embolism may be associated with cognitive deficit; therefore, patients were tested with the mini-mental status test, and auditory event related potentials were assessed testing P300 (20).

Material and methods

A total of 20 patients was recruited at random from the cardio-surgical waiting list and divided into two groups (Table 2). All patients underwent coronary artery bypass surgery with CPB under conditions of normothermia. In both groups, the heart-lung machine Stöckert S III, Cobe ECC tubing-set, Stöckert roller pump, arterial filter Cobe Sentry 21 μm, and either the Cobe CML DUO™ or Dideco D 703 Compactflo™ oxygenator equipment were used (Table 3).

Heart-lung machine priming consists of 1.0 l saline solution and 0.5 l HAES 10%.

In one group CPB was performed using an Cobe CML Duo FS™ oxygenator; in the other group a Dideco D 703 Compactflo™ was used. The measurement of high intensity signals (HITS) was performed at two different points: oxygenator inlet as well as outlet. During operation bilateral TCD monitoring (Multidop X4, DWL) was performed. Both middle cerebral arteries were insonated at two separate depths each (distal depth 44–49 mm, proximal 54–59 mm) with the patient in lying position (Fig. 2). Monitoring time was 60 minutes per patient. High intensity transients in the Doppler signal were recognized as microemboli signals (MES) based on accepted criteria (3). In brief, detection criteria were characteristic harmonic sound, intensity at least 3 db above the background, short duration, random occur-

Table 2. Patient population; oxygenator used in ECC

Oxygenator	Cobe CML DUO™	Dideco D 703 Compactflo™
Patients		
number	10	10
Age (years)	64.96+6.5	60.2+12.0
Education (years)	9.1+1.8	9.0+1.1
Sex (m/f)	m	m
NYHA	I–III	I–III

Table 3. Parameters of heart-lung machine and equipment

Parameter	Cobe CML DUO™	Dideco D 703 Compactflo™
Heart-lung machine	STÖCKERT SIII	STÖCKERT SIII
ECC tubing set	Cobe	Cobe
Arterial filter	Cobe Sentry 21 μm	Cobe Sentry 21 μm

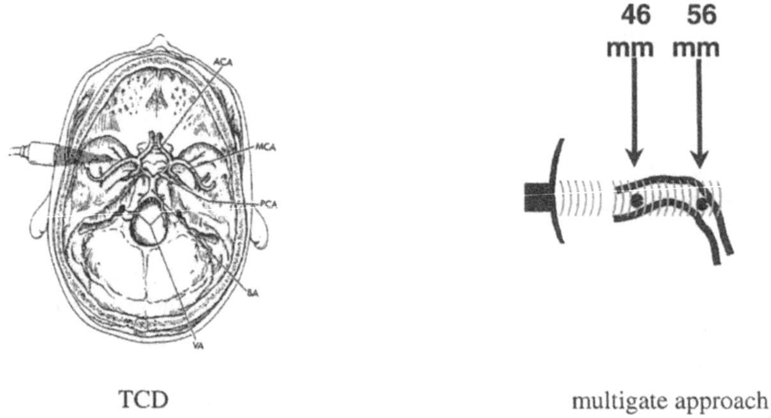

Fig. 2. Basal cerebral arteries and ultrasound probe insonating the middle cerebral artery from the transtemporal approach (left) and principle of multigate approach (right).

rence in the cardiac cycle, and time delay between the proximal and distal channels ranging from 0.02 to 0.1 seconds on subsequent spectral analysis.

Prevalence of neurological complications was evaluated on the basis of a standard neurological questionnaire (mini-mental test) and P300 testing.

Neuropsychological performance was determined before and seven days postsurgery. Performing P 300 tones were presented binaurally through headphones at an intensity of 70 dBSC. Tone bursts lasted 50 ms with 5 ms rise/fall times, with an interstimulus interval of 2.5 seconds. Target tone was 3 kHz; nontarget tone was 1.5 kHz. In order to determine the influence of rheological factors, the hematocrit, blood flow, activated clotting time (ACT), and thrombocytes were estimated (Table 4).

Table 4. Parameters of CPB and rheological data

Parameter	Cobe CML DUO™	Dideco D 703 Compactflo™
ECC time (min)	95±18.5	100.8±15.2
Operating time (h, min.)	2.56±25	3.04±13
Thrombocytes (Gpt/l)		
Pre ECC	251.8±82.2	227.0±129.9
Post ECC	163.4±59.4	130.5±54.4
Thrombodecrease (%)	−34.6±12.2	−39.1±11.1
ACT (s)	491.2±34.9	493.9±27,5
Blood flow (l/min)	5.42±0.45	5.41±0.56
Hematocrit (%)		
(minimum)	22.0±1.49	21.7±1.83
(maximum)	24.8±0.92	24.6±1.17

Table 5. MES counts (HITS/min) at oxygenator in/outlet and in TCD monitoring

Parameter	Cobe CML DUO™	Dideco D 703 Compactflo™
Oxy inlet	70.48±75.40	54.05±24.06
Oxy outlet	32.94±48,60	43.99±35.41
TCD left side	2.97±3.65	3.22±1.70
TCD right side	3.58±4.76	2.63±1.34

Table 6. Results of mini-mental and P 300 testing pre- and 7 days postsurgery

Parameter	Cobe CML DUO™	Dideco D 703 Compactflo™
P 300 (time in ms)		
Presurgery	362.90±28.86	330.78±23.48
Postsurgery	353.14±58,56	354.50±33.88
Mini-mental		
Presurgery	31.50±2.46	32.00±1.66
Postsurgery	32.29±1,80	30.89±2.47

Results

The two investigated membrane oxygenators show different numbers of counted MES at the chosen measure points. At the oxygenator inlet, the number of MES of the Cobe CML DUO is slightly higher compared to those assessed at the Dideco inlet. Otherwise, the number of assessed HITS at the oxygenator outlet is labeled by higher counts with the Dideco equipment (Table 5). The Cobe oxygenator seems to have better air trapping features.

TCD monitoring of the left and right temporal region demonstrates higher counts for the Dideco oxygenator at the left side and lower counts at the right, compared to the Cobe CML DUO, without reaching statistical significance.

Neuropsychological testing revealed no difference between the two groups prior to surgery. After surgery, in the Cobe group we obtained better results in P 300 testing (shorter latencies) as well as in the mini-mental test (Table 6). There were no significant differences in the rheological data (Table 4).

Discussion

Extracorporeal circulation (ECC) is associated with many pathophysiological changes resulting in impairment of the brain, the lungs, and kidneys (2, 12, 16). One major complication is microembolism which can cause microcirculatory obstruction. There are two kinds of microemboli, gaseous and solid particles. There is further evidence of gaseous embolic material in patients with artificial heart valves. Simultaneously performed monitoring over the middle (MCA) and anterior cerebral artery (ACA) and the common carotid artery (CCA) showed significantly higher MES counts in the CCA compared with the MCA and ACA. MES counts progressively decline with increasing distance because bubbles are bound to implode with time (5). The occurrence of gaseous embolism (air) has been markedly decreased by improvements in operating techniques and ECC equipment (oxygenator design) (19).

Three main sources of emboli are confirmed: infusion of blood stored for more than 3 days, use of cardiotomy reservoirs and oxygenators, especially bubble oxygenators (7). The tubing system of the extracorporeal circuit contains many exogenous microparticles (7, 14). After simple saline primed perfusion for ten minutes, particle counts reached values 14 times higher than before perfusion (7). Another important source of emboli is silicon oil. Roller pumps can cause a large number of particles to break off from the rubber tubes.

Membrane oxygenators are widely used because of their ability to reduce both damage to blood cells and embolism, as these types avoid direct contact of air with blood (4, 9). Microembolization is greater when bubble oxygenators are used rather than membrane oxygenators; on the other hand, the membrane oxygenator is the site for most of the thrombus formation, subjected to repeated periods of unclamping and clamping to direct blood flow. We detected microemboli with Doppler ultrasound, using the bigate approach in TCD as a new tool for investigating embolization. Ultrasound cannot detect particles smaller than 50 μm and is, thus, more sensitive to air bubbles than to solid emboli.

In our study, the cognitive deficits assessed postsurgery are associated with the type of oxygenator used in the CPB circuit. Our results show the tendency that the degree of neurological damage (depressed neuropsychometric test scores) is related to number and size of microemboli. Agreeing with the studies of other authors, the left side of cerebral circulation seems to be more susceptible for brain injury due to microembolism (10, 14). Microembolism due to the ECC circuit may effect cognitive function. The P 300 test may be a sensitive additional procedure to assess cognitive deficits. Prolonged P 300 latency is an indicator of disturbed information processing in the brain. Cognitive deficits before and increased disturbation after cardiac surgery suggest vulnerability of patients with already compromised cerebral function (17). Therefore, most recent data justify further evaluation of the influence of the CPB equipment and promise benefit for the cognitive outcome (decrease neuropsychiatric abnormalities after CPB), especially of neurologically compromised patients.

References

1. Andrew MJ, Baker RA, Kneebone AC, Knight JL (1998) Neuropsychological dysfunction after minimally invasive direct coronary artery bypass grafting. Ann Thorac Surg 66:1611–1617
2. Babin-Ebell J, Misoph M, Mullges W, Neukam K, Reese J, Elert O (1999) Intraoperative embolus formation during cardiopulmonary bypass affects the release of S100B. Thorac Cardiovasc Surg. 47:166–169
3. Consensus Committee of the Ninth International Cerebral Hemodynamics Symposium (1995) Basic identification criteria of Doppler microemboli signals. Stroke 26:1123
4. De Jong JCF, ten Duis HJ, Smit Sibinga CT, Wildevuur CRH (1980) Hematotopic aspects of cardiotomy suction in cardiac operations. J Thorac Cardiovasc Surg 79:227–236
5. Georgiadis D, Baumgartner RW, Karatschai R, Lindner A, Zerkowski H-R (1998) Further evidence of gaseous embolic material in patients with artificial heart valves. J Thorac Cardiovasc Surg 115:808–810
6. Georgiadis D, Preiß M, Lindner A, Gybels Y, Zierz S, Zerkowski H-R (1997) Doppler microembolic signals in children with prosthetic cardiac valves. Stroke 28(7):1328–1329
7. Jin-Feng Lin, Zhao-Kang Su, Wen-Xiang Ding (1992) Quantitation of particulate microemboli during cardiopulmonary bypass: Experimental and clinical studies. Ann Thorac Surg 54:1196–1202
8. Kenneth M, Taylor MD (1998) Brain damage during cardiopulmonary bypass. Ann Thorac Surg 65:20–26
9. Nishida H, Aomi S, Tomizawa Y, Endo M, Koyanagi H, Nojiri Oshiyama H, Kido T, Yokoyama K (1999) Comparative study of biocompatibility between the open circuit and closed circuit in cardiopulmonary bypass. Artif Organs 47:547–551
10. Orenstein JM, Sato N, Aaron B et al (1982) Microemboli observed in deaths following cardiopulmonary bypass surgery: silicone antifoam agents and polyvinylchloride tubing as source of emboli. Hum Pathol 13:1082–1090
11. Padayachee TS, Parsons S, Theobold R, Linley J, Gosling RG, Deverall PB (1987) The detection of microemboli in the middle cerebral artery during cardiopulmonary bypass: a transcranial Doppler ultrasound investigation using membrane and bubble oxygenators. Ann Thorac Surg 44:298–302
12. Ratliff NB, Young WG Jr, Hackel BB et al (1973) Pulmonary injury secondary to extracorporeal circulation. J Thorac Cardiovasc Surg 65:425–432
13. Shaw PJ, Bates D, Cartlidge NE, Heaviside D, Julian DG, Shaw DA (1985) Early neurological complications of coronary artery bypass surgery. Br Med J 291:1384–1387
14. Fink SM, Bockman DE, Howell CG, Falls DG, Kanto WP Jr (1989) Bypass circuits as the source of thromboembolism during extracorporeal membrane oxygenation. J Pediatr 115:621–624
15. Sylivris S, Levi C, Matalanis G, Rosalion A, Buxton BF, Mitchell A, Fitt G, Harberts DB, Saling MM, Tonkin AM (1998) Pattern and significance of cerebral microemboli during coronary artery bypass grafting. Ann Thorac Surg 66:1674–1678
16. Taylor RL, Borger MA, Weisel RD, Fedorko L, Feindel CM (1999) Cerebral microemboli during cardiopulmonary bypass: increased emboli during perfusionist interventions. Ann Thorac Surg 68:89–93
17. Toner I, Taylor KM, Newman S, PLC-Smith (1998) Cerebral function changes following cardiac surgery: Neuropsychological and EEG assessment. Eur J Cardiothorac Surg 13:13–20
18. Van der Linden J, Casimir-Ahn H (1991) When do cerebral emboli appear during open heart operations? A transcranial Doppler study. Ann Thorac Surg 51:237–241
19. Wimmer-Greinecker G, Matheis G, Martens S, Oremek G, Abdel-Rahman U, Moritz A (1999) Synthetic protein treated versus heparin coated cardiopulmonary bypass surfaces: similar clinical results and minor biochemical differences. Eur J Cardiothorac Surg 16:211-217

20. Chen Y-J, Kang W-M, Warren CH-M So (1996) Comparison of antiepileptic drugs on cognitive function in newly diagnosed epileptic children: A psychometric and neuropsychological study. Epilepsia 37:81–86

Author's address:
Prof. Dr. H.-R. Zerkowski
Klinik für Herz- und Thoraxchirurgie
Universitätsklinik
Kantonsspital Basel
Spitalstr. 21
CH-4031 Basel, Schweiz

S100B as a diagnostic tool for brain damage after cardiac surgery

H. Jönsson
Department of Cardiothoracic Surgery, University Hospital, Lund, Sweden

Background

Cerebral complications are a major cause of morbidity after cardiac surgery. Ischemic stroke with neurological deficits can be very disabling for the patient, e.g., when the localization of the ischemia results in a hemiparesis. Whereas a minor ischemic lesion or a lesion with a more favorable localization does give such devastating symptoms. Still the incidence of a stroke, i.e., a regional ischemia with neurological symptoms, after cardiac surgery has been reported to occur between 0.7–5.2% (Lynn et al., 1985).

The diagnosis of an ischemic stroke relies on clinical examination and radiological methods, such as computed tomography (CT) or magnetic resonance imaging (MRI). These methods give either a functional or an anatomical diagnosis of consequences of regional ischemia.

The most common neurological complication is however not the stroke, but a subtle cognitive dysfunction. This is a complication with a reduction in cognitive function, such as memory function, ability to learn new task, and abstract thinking, and it occurs in up to 79% of patients (9). Many patients perceive difficulties in small everyday tasks, like learning a telephone number or remembering what to buy when they go to the convenience store.

To diagnose a cognitive dysfunction after cardiac surgery is difficult. At present the cognitive dysfunction is measured with neuropsychological tests; no other method has shown to be as useful. Neuropsychological tests have some drawbacks: they are time consuming since they require a preoperative base-line test and 1–2 post-operative tests and each test takes approximately one hour. Also, these tests are best performed by a trained tester, such as a neuropsychologist. The inherited difficulties with the test makes a routine testing of all patients a cumbersome task, and to date these tests have only been used in research.

Other new methods to diagnose a post-operative neurological complication have been suggested, e.g., cerebral blood flow (CBF), trans-cranial doppler (TCD) and biochemical markers. Many of these techniques have methodological problems, for instance, some of the suggested biochemical markers have only been found in cerebrospinal fluid (CSF). However, lately S100B has been suggested as a promising marker, and it can be found in peripheral blood after cardiac surgery.

S100B Protein

S100B is a protein that is abundant in brain tissue, especially in glial and Schwann cells. The protein is a dimer, combined from the two subunits, S100A and S100B (7). The two dimers are S100A1B and S100BB. It is the B-subunit which is brain specific and is measured by the available assays, whereas the α-subunit is present in high concentrations in many tissues and therefore lacks in organ specificity. S100B is also present in other tissues besides brain, but in low concentrations. The tissue with the second highest concentration after brain is fat, which has 2.8–5.5% of the concentration in brain tissue (4).

S100B have been shown to have both extra- and intra-cellular effects. Extracellularly, it can act both neurotoxic and neuroprotective. Intracellularly, S100B acts as a calcium-binding protein; intracellular calcium is bound to S100B at specific calcium sites on the protein. The S100B-calcium complex then binds to a different effector protein, which can exert a specific effect, such as regulation of cell structure, energy metabolism or learning.

S100B is not normally found in serum, but after different types of brain damage, increased levels in serum have been detected. In global anoxia after cardiac arrest, S100B seems to reflect the severity of ischemia and the level has a predictive value on outcome after such an event (10). S100B levels have also been shown to correlate with size of infarction after stroke in patients admitted to the emergency room and predict functional status in these patients after the stroke (3). S100B has also been shown to be useful in determining the severity of the brain trauma in patients presenting with a minor head injury (MHI).

S100 in cardiac surgery

Given the high incidence of cerebral morbidity after cardiac surgery and the suboptimal diagnostic tests available, a biochemical marker, like S100B, is desirable, since there are obvious advantages with a biochemical marker. For instance, sampling of blood for analysis of S100B can be performed any specific time in relation to imposed surgical trauma, and a quick analysis of S100B levels could give the clinician an indication that brain damage is evolving, and open an opportunity to intervene.

The present studies on S100 have focused on patients undergoing surgery with cardiopulmonary bypass (CPB), and the knowledge of so-called "off-pump surgery" is limited. In patients undergoing surgery with CPB, S100B is not present in blood before surgery; it starts to increase during surgery and peaks at the end of surgery. Increased levels are found in almost all patients the first few hours after surgery, 13% of patients have increased levels 48 hours after surgery, and in some patients a persistent release is found up to 4 days after surgery.

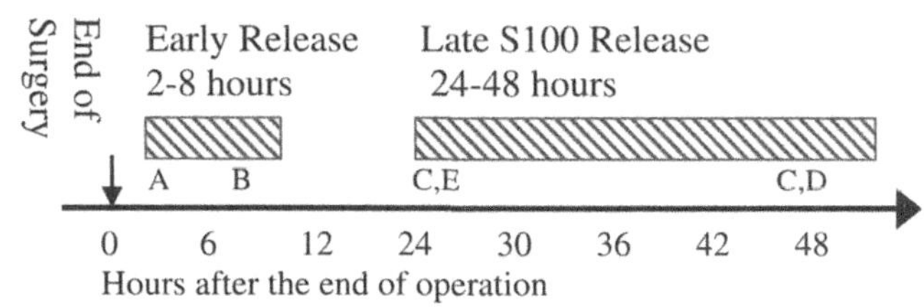

Fig. 1. Early and late release of S100B after cardiac surgery together with times for important findings. End of surgery defined as termination of perfusion with heart-lung machine. (A) In a study of 90 patients, an association between S100B levels 1–4 hours after surgery and neuropsychological outcome was found. (B) In a study of 130 patients, higher S100B levels were found 7 hours after surgery in the group who performed worse on memory test. (C) In a study of 27 patients, 4 patients developed stroke and had increased S100B values 24 and 48 hours after surgery. (D) In a study of 515 patients, 13 patients with a postoperative stroke had increased levels 48 hours after surgery. (E) In a series of eight patients with a postoperative stroke, a strong correlation was found between size of the brain infarction and S100B serum levels.

Early and late S100β release

In cardiac surgery the release of S100B can be divided into an early release which occurs the first few hours after surgery and a late release which occurs 24–48 (96) hours after surgery (Fig. 1).

The late release is associated with an ischemic event (see below) and probably depends on a release from dying glial cells in combination of a corrupted Blood-brain barrier (BBB).

The early release measured the first few hours after surgery comes from at least two different sources. First, an extracerebral source has been identified which obscures S100B levels the first few hours immediately after surgery and second, a release from the brain, whose origin is unclear. However, it has been speculated that it could be a washout of extracellular S100B when the integrity of the BBB has been compromised as a consequence of the extracorporeal circulation.

S100B kinetics

To fully understand how measurements of serum S100B concentrations after cardiac surgery can be used, we must look into the kinetics of this protein. Like any other protein or drug, the kinetics of S100B depend mainly on 3 different factors: first, the release or infusion of S100B into the circulation; second, the distribution of the protein in the circulation; and third, the elimination of the protein. These three factors are all important in understanding S100B kinetics after cardiac surgery and will therefore be explained.

Brain release and extracerebral contamination of S100B

S100B is a highly brain-specific protein, and an increase in serum levels have therefore been assumed to be of cerebral origin. However, in the case of cardiac surgery an extracerebral source has been identified. All shed blood collected from the surgical field contains high levels of S100B (6). It is routine practice to collect shed mediastinal during surgery by cardiotomy suction and return it to the patient through the heart-lung machine. In the postoperative period, shed mediastinal blood is also collected, and many cardiac surgery units retransfuse this blood to the patient by means of autotransfusion. Since this collected shed blood contains high levels of S100B, a concurrent increase in serum levels of S100B is seen after the retransfusion of this shed blood, as illustrated in Fig. 2. This increase does not reflect a cerebral release, but instead obscures the cerebral release. This extracerebral S100B probably originates from a breakdown of adipose tissue in the surgical field. Other adipocyte-specific substances, like hormone-sensitive lipase, have also been found in the shed blood, indicating a breakdown of adipocytes. If this contamination of S100B is excluded, i.e., no collected shed blood is retransfused, a cerebral release is found the first few hours after surgery, as illustrated in Fig. 3.

If S100B originating from the brain is found in peripheral blood, it must have passed the BBB, whose integrity is compromised. The BBB can be opened by, for instance, ischemia, inflammatory response, hyperosmolar solutions or toxic agents. Probably some of these mechanisms act to open the BBB during cardiac surgery. With an open BBB S100B can be released either from intra- or extra-cellular deposits in the brain and enter the circulation.

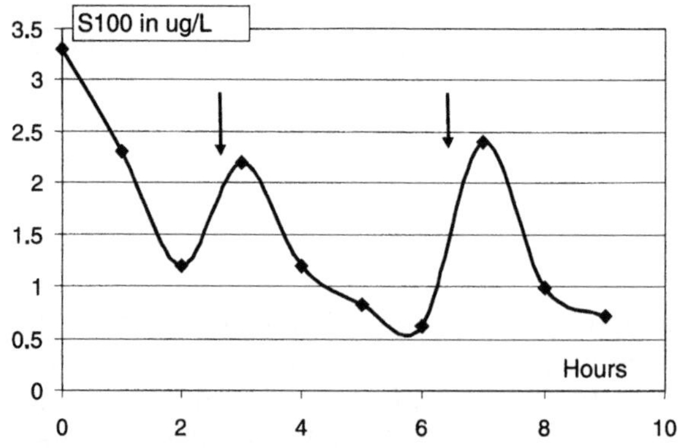

Fig. 2. Serum levels of S100B in a CABG patient who received shed mediastinal blood during surgery and intermittent autotransfusion after surgery (arrows). Hours denote time after the termination of cardiopulmonary bypass with the heart lung machine.

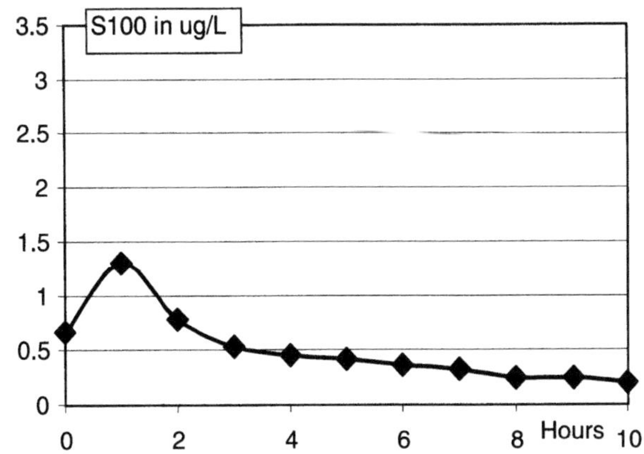

Fig. 3. Serum levels of S100B in a CABG patient where the collected shed blood during surgery was processed in cell-saver device and where no autotransfusion was given.

Distribution of protein

S100B is 21 Kda protein and does not pass an intact vascular endothelium. The distribution volume after cardiac surgery has been determined to be 8.8 liters, which is just a little bit more than the blood volume (6). Therefore, S100B follows the distribution pattern of other proteins and does not undergo any significant redistribution to other compartments besides blood after cardiac surgery.

Elimination of S100B

Like other proteins in this range, e.g., β2-microglobulin, S100B is believed to be eliminated by the kidneys by means of degradation in the distal tubuli. The biological half-life has been determined to 25 min and follows a first order kinetics (submitted). This quick elimination indicates two things: first, if increased levels of S100B can be measured in serum, there is an ongoing release. Second, a contamination, such as the infusion of shed blood, is cleared within 5 half-lives (2 hours), since after 5 half-lives only $1/32^{nd}$ of the contamination is left. These low residual levels of the contamination do not interfere with the cerebral S100B.

In conclusion, extracerebral contamination of serum S100B levels is caused by infusion of shed blood. Since S100B has a short half-life, this extracerebral contamination is eliminated within 2 hours after the last administration. If autotransfusion is not used in the postoperative care of the patients, the contamination of S100B from shed blood during surgery is cleared 2 hours after the termination of CPB. This is illustrated in Fig. 4, where the S100B levels immediately after surgery have been assumed to only have extracerebral origin and, with a half-life of 25 min, this extracerebral is

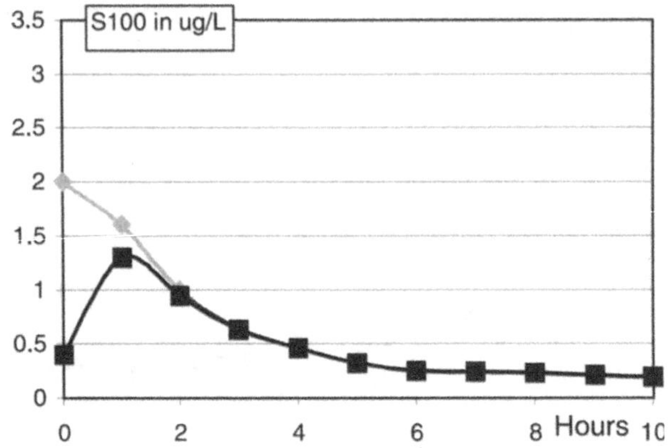

Fig. 4. The measured S100B levels (◆) in a CABG patient together with the calculated true cerebral levels (■), where extracerebral levels have been excluded by a kinetic calculation.

eliminated in 2 hours and levels measured after that reflect cerebral release. If, however, autotransfusion is used, the cerebral S100B is obscured up to two hours after the end of administration.

Late S100B release

Late S100B release, defined as 1 to 2 days after surgery, has been related to a postoperative stroke in several studies (Fig. 1). In a study of 515 coronary artery bypass graft patients, 13 developed stroke and these patients also had elevated S100B levels 15 and 48 hours after surgery (5). The studies presented on S100B and stroke have only looked into S100B levels between 15 and 48 hours after surgery. However, in stroke patients presenting to the emergency room, increased levels have been found up to 5 days after the stroke. It can, therefore, be assumed that in cardiac surgery increased levels of S100B are found between 1 and 5 days, like the example of a patient with a postoperative stroke presented in Fig. 5. Preliminary findings also show a correlation between S100B concentration 24 hours after surgery and size of the ischemic lesion, as illustrated in Fig. 6. This is a finding which supports the theory that S100B is more a marker of amount of damaged brain tissue than a marker for functional outcome.

In the material presented so far it has not been possible to make a clear cut-off point for S100B. Eighty seven percent of patients without symptoms of a postoperative stroke do not have detectable S100B levels 48 hours after surgery. Thus, 13% of patients without symptoms still have increased S100B levels, the reason for this is unclear but silent ischemia, i.e., infarcted brain tissue without neurological symptoms, could explain some of the 13%.

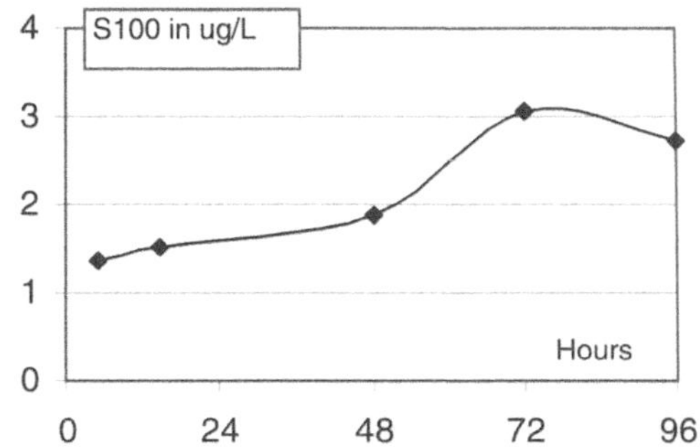

Fig. 5. Example of serum S100B levels in a 68 year old patient who suffered postoperative stroke. The patient had a stroke 2 years before and underwent a CABGx5. After surgery, he developed bilateral paresis, with improvement of right side, and a severe dysphasia. CT at 3 days and MRI at 17 showed infarctions in the cerebellum, brain stem, bilateral in occipital and periventricular white matter.

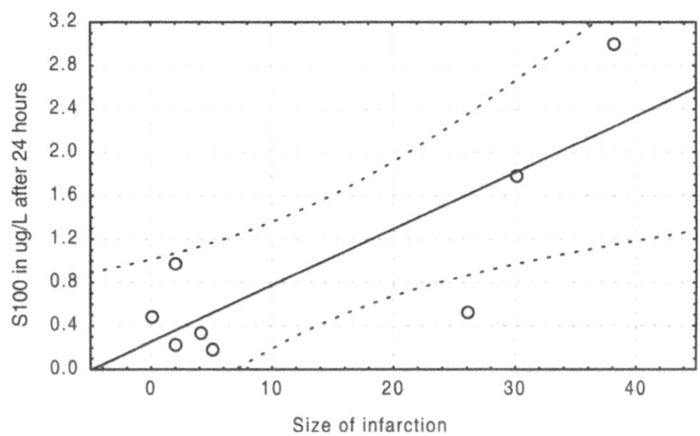

Fig. 6. The relation between size of infarcted area, measured with a semiquantitative method from CT-scans, and S100B levels 24 hours after surgery in 8 patients who suffered a post-operative stroke ($r=0.76$, $p<0.05$).

Another interesting finding is that patients with atheroma of the ascending aorta, which is a well-known risk factor for post-operative stroke, and without an overt stroke have increased S100B levels 48 hours after surgery. This finding suggests that there may be a considerable number of patients who suffer silent ischemia after surgery as detected by S100B but without symptoms of neurological deficits.

From the available material, we can however deduce that a serum S100B level above 0.5 µg/L 24 or 48 hours after surgery is associated with a large brain infarction with gross neurological deficits and is seen on computed tomography (CT).

The origin of the late S100B release is unclear. To be able to speculate on the origin, we must recollect some of the mechanisms found in cerebral ischemia.

A few minutes of cerebral ischemia starts the ischemic cascade, which starts with a large inflow of calcium into the cells and eventually leads to cellular death after 24 hours. The cell death can be due to depletion of oxygen and glucose or by cellular apoptosis. The end-stage of this cascade is a disruption of cellular membranes, which makes the intracellular proteins flow freely out to the extracellular space. Since S100B is present in a much higher concentration intracellularly than extracellularly, this would raise the concentration of S100B in the extracellular matrix, and together with an open BBB this could be the mechanism for the increase of S100B detected in blood.

Also there is an area around the core of the infarction called the penumbra region. The penumbra can be hypoxic for several days with viable neurons and glial cells, and a protracted cellular death is often seen in this area, which could explain that high S100B levels are found several days after the insult.

It is therefore reasonable to assume that the late S100B increase seen after a post-operative stroke is from intracellular S100B in dead cells which have ruptured.

Early S100B release

The early release of S100B, defined as 2 to 8 hours after surgery, is more difficult to understand both when it comes to origin and its relation to neurological morbidity.

The origin of early S100B release is probably not from intracellular deposits, since disruption of cell walls takes longer and any mechanisms for release of S100B into the extracellular matrix are not known. Instead, it is more likely that the BBB opens, due to either the inflammatory response or any other exogenous factor from the heart-lung machine, which makes diffusion of matrix proteins like S100B over the BBB possible. An extracellular source, alone or together with a possible upregulation of S100B synthesis, is the suggested mechanism for early S100B release.

The early release of S100B has been found to be associated with a cognitive dysfunction in a couple of studies (Fig. 1). However, the extracerebral contamination has not been taken into account in one of these studies, which makes the interpretation of these data a bit haphazardous. These studies do, however, point out an interesting connection between a biochemical event and behavioral change like the decline in cognitive dysfunction.

The time interval suggested for the early release is based on the fact that it takes 2 hours to clear the contamination of S100B from shed blood during surgery, and after approximately 8 hours the levels found in serum have declined in most patients to levels around the detection limit (Fig. 4).

S100B in research

In research there is a need for a new tool to measure neurological morbidity after cardiac surgery. Studies that compare surgical techniques and other studies aimed at reducing neurological complications need an objective, simple and easily interpreted end-point. The presented results on S100B indicate that S100B could be such an end-point. In fact, measurements of S100B levels have been used in a couple studies to compare different surgical techniques.

A comparison between bypass circuit with and without an arterial line filter showed small differences between the groups 5 and 24 hours after surgery, where the group with the arterial line filter had lower S100B levels. The earlier S100B levels, at the end of surgery, did not differ between groups (12, 13).

Coronary artery bypass surgery was also compared to intracardiac surgery, such as valve and septum defects surgery, with S100B as the only end-point. Higher S100B levels were found 5 and 24 hours after surgery in the intracardiac surgery group than in the coronary artery bypass group. In this study one patient presented with a post-operative stroke and had increased levels after 24 hours (12, 13).

A strong relation between the time of circulatory arrest and S100B levels 1 day after surgery in patients who underwent surgery with hypothermic arrest was found (1). This finding is interesting because the longer period of circulatory arrest with cerebral ischemia, the greater the risk for neuronal death. An increase 24 hours after surgery therefore indicates a glial cell breakdown as a result of a prolonged ischemia. Even though patients with circulatory arrest go through surgery without signs of regional ischemia, such as stroke, the global ischemia may lead to a diffuse cell death.

Discussion

Undoubtedly there is a need, both in clinical practice and in research, for a simple method of measuring any cerebral complication after cardiac surgery. A screening method for ischemic lesions after surgery, which can detect an ischemic lesion that does not present with overt neurological deficits, and therefore may pass unnoticed, is needed.

Also, a simpler method that could be used for diagnosis and prediction of cognitive dysfunction is desired. The method of choice today to make such a diagnosis requires 2–3 prospective neuropsychological tests. A simpler method to be used in screening of all patients, and also used as an end-point in research aimed at reducing neurological complications, would therefore be very useful.

A biochemical marker meets some of these demands since it is easy to use, inexpensive, and objective. If the biochemical marker could be shown to have high sensitivity and specificity in the diagnosis of ischemic lesions and cognitive dysfunction, it would have a given position in clinical practice and research.

S100B have shown interesting results and could be the biochemical marker that fulfills these requirements. One methodological problem with this marker is the extracerebral contamination from shed mediastinal blood. However, with the kinetic information presented, this can be overcome with proper sampling times.

The late release after 1 day and later is associated with a postoperative stroke. Hopefully, further studies will show more clearly that the levels of S100B correlate with size and clinical outcome. In patients with stroke admitted to the emergency room, the higher the S100B levels, the larger the infarction and the worse the outcome. This will probably be shown to be valid for patients undergoing cardiac surgery as well.

The early release has been associated with cognitive dysfunction. However, several methodological problems are found in this field. First, cognitive dysfunction is measured with a neuropsychological test, which gives a functional assessment of the brain. We do not know anything about the underlying biochemical processes behind the decline in cognitive function. Second, neuropsychological tests are not easily interpreted; several definitions of decline are present and methodological problems, e.g., regression to the mean, make the results of these tests sometimes difficult to interpret. Third, the extracerebral S100B can obscure true cerebral release. In some of the studies published on S100B, contamination was not taken into account; therefore, the results are biased and probably underestimated the strength of the association between S100B and outcome.

Hopefully, future research will clarify some of these methodological problems and explore the potential strength of S100B as a biochemical marker for cognitive dysfunction after cardiac surgery. In the case of a post-operative stroke, S100B levels have shown clearer results for its feasibility to detect a stroke, thus, giving it a place in everyday clinical practice.

References

1. Astudillo R, Van der Linden J, Radegran K, Hansson L-O, Åberg B (1996) Elevated serum levels of S-100 after deep hypothermic arrest correlate with duration of circulatory arrest. Eur J Cardiothorac Surg 10:1107–1113
2. Blomquist S, Johnsson P, Lührs C, Malmkvist G, Solem J-O, Alling C et al (1997) The appearence of S-100 protein in serum during and immediately after cardiopulmonary bypass surgery. A possible marker for cerebral injury. J Cardiothorac Vasc Anesth 11:699–703
3. Büttner T, Weyers S, Postert T, Sprengelmeyer R, Kuhn W (1997) S-100 protein: Serum marker of focal brain damage after ischemic territorial MCA infarction. Stroke 28:1961–1965
4. Haimoto H, Hosoda S, Kato K (1987) Differential distribution of immunoreactive S100-alpha and S100-beta proteins in normal nonnervous human tissues. Lab Invest 57(5):489–498

5. Jönsson H, Johnsson P, Alling C, Westaby S, Blomquist S (1998) Significance of serum S100 release after coronary artery surgery. Ann Thorac Surg
6. Jönsson H, Johnsson P, Alling C, Bäckström M, Bergh C, Blomquist S (in press) S100B after coronary artery surgery: release pattern, source of contamination and relation to neuropsychological outcome. Ann Thorac Surg
7. Kligman D, Hilt DC (1988) The S100 protein family. Trends Biochem Sci 13(11):437–443
8. Lynn GM, Stefanko K, Reed JF (1992) Risk factors for stroke after coronary artery bypass. J Thorac Cardiovasc Surg 104:1518–1523
9. Mahanna EP, Blumenthal JA, White WD, Croughwell ND, Clancy CP, Smith LR et al (1996) Defining neuropsychological dysfunction after coronary artery bypass grafting. Ann Thorac Surg 61:1342–1347
10. Rosen H, Rosengren L, Herlitz J, Blomstrand C (1998) Increased serum levels of the S-100 protein are associated with hypoxic brain damage after cardiac arrest. Stroke 29:473–477
11. Sandström E, Svenmarker S, Karlsson K, Åberg T (1996) S-100 and memory function after cardiac surgery. European association of cardiothoracic surgery, meeting Prague
12. Taggart DP, Bhattacharya K, Meston N, Standing S, Kay J, Pillai R et al (1997) Serum S-100 protein concentration after cardiac surgery: a randomized trial of arterial line filtration. Eur J Cardiothorac Surg 11:645–649
13. Taggart DP, Mazel JW, Bhattacharya K, Meston N, Standing SJ, Kay JD et al (1997) Comparison of serum S-100 beta levels during CABG and intracardiac operations. Ann Thorac Surg 63(2):492–496
14. Zimmer DB, Cornwall EH, Landar A, Song W (1995) The S100 protein family: history, function, and expression. Brain Res Bull 37(4):417–429

Author's address:
Henrik Jönsson, M.D.
Thoraxkirurgiska Kliniken
Universitetssjukhuset
SE-22185 Lund, Sweden

Pathophysiological predictors of the short- and long-term neurobehavioral outcome of cardiac surgery with extracorporeal circulation

M. Herrmann[1], Ch. Huth[2], and A.D. Ebert[1]
[1] Division of Neuropsychology and Behavioral Neurology, Otto-von-Guericke-University, Magdeburg, Germany
[2] Department of Thoracic and Cardiovascular Surgery, Otto-von-Guericke-University, Magdeburg, Germany

Introduction

Neurobehavioral sequelae of cardiac surgery under cardiopulmonary bypass conditions have gained increasing importance during the last few decades. There are several lines of arguments which demonstrate the significance of neurobehavioral alterations after heart surgery; four of them will be outlined in the following:

- Although cardiac surgery has become much safer when judged by the incidence rates of adverse neurological outcome, the figures for subtle neurobehavioral alterations remain high. Depending on the respective neuropsychological test procedures, the time of assessment, and the patient groups involved, incidence data of postoperative neuropsychological deficits range up to 80% (10) with a peak incidence of about 30%.
- Neurobehavioral disorders after cardiac surgery cause additional costs for inpatient treatment and rehabilitation. Roach and coworkers (12) estimated an additional $6,150 in-hospital boarding costs for patients with postoperative neurobehavioral disorders. This figure, however, does not include the increased spending caused by rehabilitation or early retirement due to persisting neuropsychological deficits.
- Obviously, neurobehavioral disorders have a major impact on the postoperative quality of life of patients undergoing cardiac surgery under cardiopulmonary bypass conditions. Research on variables influencing the short- and long-term neurobehavioral outcome may, therefore, help to improve the overall benefit of cardiac surgery.
- In contrast to patient groups which are usually subject of neuropsychological research, the prevailing number of patients undergoing cardiac surgery with extracorporeal circulation show no substantial preoperative brain disorders. Heart surgery under cardiopulmonary bypass conditions, therefore, represents a unique paradigm of "experimental brain research in humans" (also named as "virtual laboratory of delirium research" by Heller and Kornfeld (4)) which may provide valuable insight into the pathophysiology of neuropsychological disorders.

Neurobehavioral disorders – definition of the term and incidence rates

During the last few decades, psychological alterations after cardiac surgery have been described with a variety of different definitions. The most often used terms were "psycho-organic syndrome", "postoperative delirium", "acute cerebral dysfunction" or "psychologic alterations" (compare (17)). None of these terms, however, is based on an operational definition and some of the descriptions imply a transitional character of postoperative psychological disorders which very often did not apply to the long-lasting neuropsychological deficits. More recently, the term "neurobehavioral disorders" was established. This term, on the one hand, refers to a brain disorder as the obvious cause of behavioral dysfunction and, on the other hand, combines neuropsychiatric and neuropsychological disorders. Figure 1 shows a selective synopsis of neuropsychiatric and neuropsychological disorders which form part of neurobehavioral alterations as a consequence of heart surgery with cardiopulmonary bypass. Neuropsychiatric disorders are usually presented during the first two to five days after surgery and cover a variety of psychiatric symptoms. Neuropsychological disorders include a broad range of cognitive changes, the majority of which are only detectable in detailed neuropsychological investigations (9). A more recent review by Selnes and colleagues (14) stated that not all neurobehavioral changes can be attributed to heart surgery and some of the short-term neuropsychological alterations may also accompany other surgical procedures. But especially memory and visuospatial deficits, which could last several years, might be caused by hypoperfusion, hypoxia or microemboli due to cardiopulmonary bypass. These pathophysiological conditions predominantly affect the posterior borderzone area of cerebral vascular supply particularly vulnerable to hypoxia (see next section: Vulnerability to neurobehavioral disorders).

Figure 2 shows incidence data of neurobehavioral disorders from recent studies by our group. Eight of 100 patients undergoing valve replacement and/or coronary artery bypass grafting exhibited a delirium at the postacute

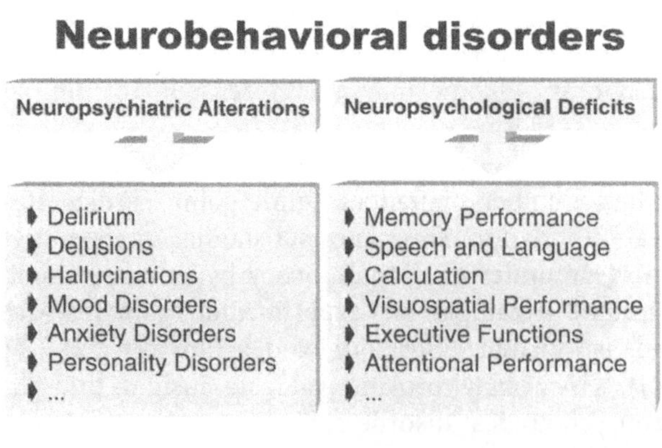

Fig. 1. Synopsis of selected neurobehavioral disorders after cardiac surgery.

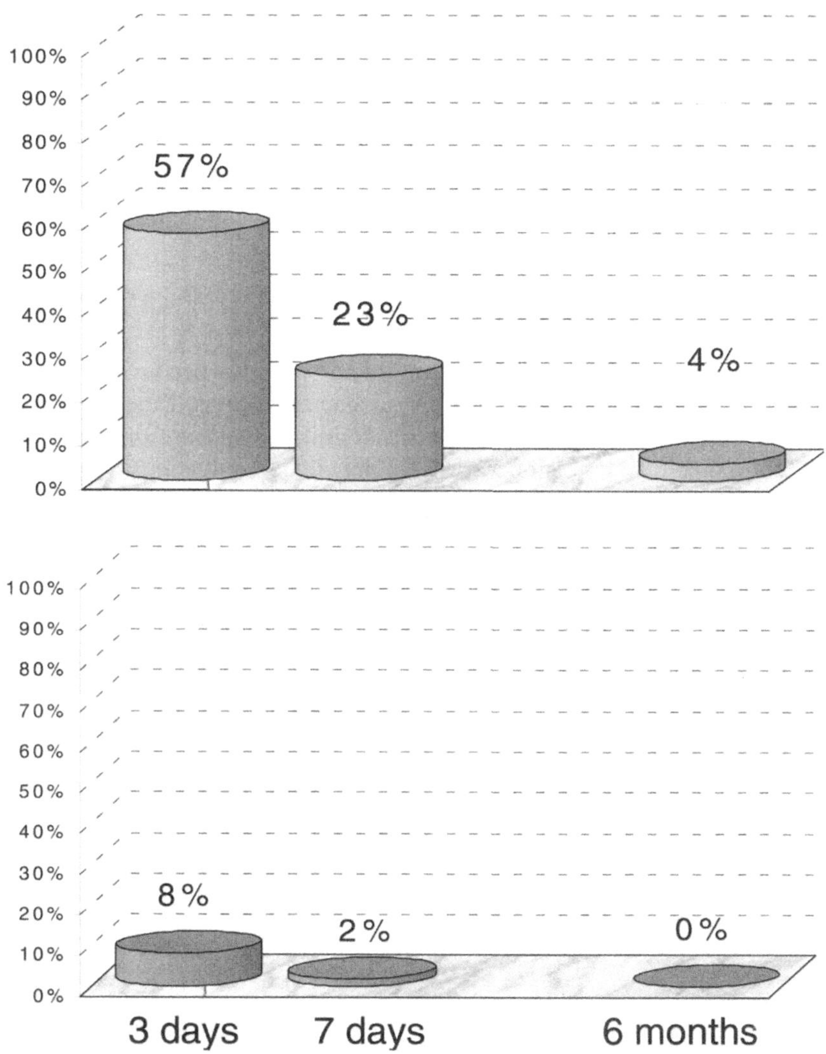

Fig. 2. Incidence rates of neurobehavioral disorders 2 and 7 days and half a year after surgery (neuropsychological disorders (top) and delirium according to DSM-III R criteria (bottom)). Neuropsychological disorder is defined as a performance more than 1.5 standard deviations below the preoperative level in at least 3 neuropsychological domains.

stage after surgery but one week after surgery only 2 patients showed a delirious disorder according to DSM-III R criteria. The figure for neuropsychological deficits, however, was far above the incidence rate for neuropsychiatric disorders. Neuropsychological disorders were operationally defined by the use of statistical criteria: All patients who scored more than 1.5 standard deviations below their respective preoperative performance in at least 3 neuropsychological domains were defined as exhibiting neuropsychological disorders. According to these harsh criteria, 57% and 23% of the patients, respectively, presented neuropsychological disorders during the first week after surgery. Six months later, the incidence data – defined by the same criteria – dropped to 4%. The use of softer criteria (e.g., deficits in only 2 neuropsychological domains) leads to an increase to 24% of patients with neuropsychological disorders half a year after surgery.

Vulnerability to neurobehavioral disorders after cardiac surgery

There is a large amount of literature on the possible predictors of neurologic and neurobehavioral disorders after cardiac operations. Due to extremely different study designs and methods, no definite conclusion on the significance of pre-, intra-, and postoperative factors affecting the postoperative neuropsychological state can be drawn so far. Figure 3 shows a selection of vari-

Preoperative Stage:

- age,
- preoperative cognitive state,
- history of cardiac, neurologic or psychiatric diseases,
- proximal aortic arteriosclerosis,
- drug treatment,
- drug or alcohol withdrawal,
- personality traits,
- ...

Intraoperative Stage:

- type of surgery,
- cross clamp time,
- hypotension,
- hypothermia,
- pulsatile vs. non-pulsatile flow,
- type of oxygenator,
- macro-/ micro-embolia
- ...

Postoperative Stage:

- length of intubation,
- sensory- / sleep deprivation,
- hyperstimulation,
- length of stay on ICU,
- postoperative complications,
- ...

Fig. 3. Selected variables affecting the neurobehavioral outcome of cardiac surgery under cardiopulmonary bypass conditions.

ables which might be associated with an adverse neuropsychological outcome after heart surgery. There is convergent evidence that a history of neurologic disease and alcohol abuse, advanced age (combined with a lower preoperative cognitive performance (18) and a higher degree of atherosclerosis), length of cross clamp or perfusion time, and type of oxygenator are those variables which explain the most significant portion of the postoperative decrease of neuropsychological functions. Furthermore, the majority of studies comparing the type of surgery under cardiopulmonary bypass condition reported patients undergoing valve replacement to be more vulnerable for neurobehavioral disorders compared to patients with coronary artery bypass grafting. A retrospective study (7) reported more frequent neurologic disorders in isolated bypass (CABG) than in valve replacement (VR) surgery. The authors attributed this finding to a world-wide increasing age of patients presenting for CABG surgery. This fact demonstrates that the majority of factors influencing the vulnerability of postoperative neurobehavioral complications are confounded. Patients with advanced age obviously have a higher probability of neurologic diseases and a higher risk for atherosclerosis and/or a possible predementia process. Studies, however, which control for well known risk factors are extremely rare.

Neurobehavioral disorders after valve replacement and coronary artery bypass grafting

During the last five years we conducted 3 studies which aimed at a comparison of neurobehavioral disorders in the postacute stage after cardiac surgery in patients undergoing either isolated coronary bypass or valve replacement surgery. In order to control for well-known risk factors, both patient samples were strictly matched for age, sex, and the preoperative neuropsychological performance. The first study (19) investigated the neuropsychological performance of 20 patients with elective valve replacement surgery and 20 patients with routine coronary artery bypass surgery. All patients were investigated preoperatively, 2 to 3 and 5 to 9 days postoperatively with the Mini-Mental-State Examination and a comprehensive neuropsychological assessment including orientation, word fluency, naming, calculation, memory, and visuospatial tasks. The results show that both groups of patients exhibit a significant early postoperative impairment of cognitive functions. Whereas the group of coronary artery bypass patients reached the preoperative level at the one week postoperative investigation, patients undergoing valve replacement surgery exhibited significantly more severe and significantly more persistent neuropsychological deficits. Postoperative neuropsychological dysfunction was mostly marked in verbal fluency and memory tasks (see Fig. 4).

In a more recent study we investigated the preoperative and short- and long-term postoperative neuropsychological performance in 46 patients un-

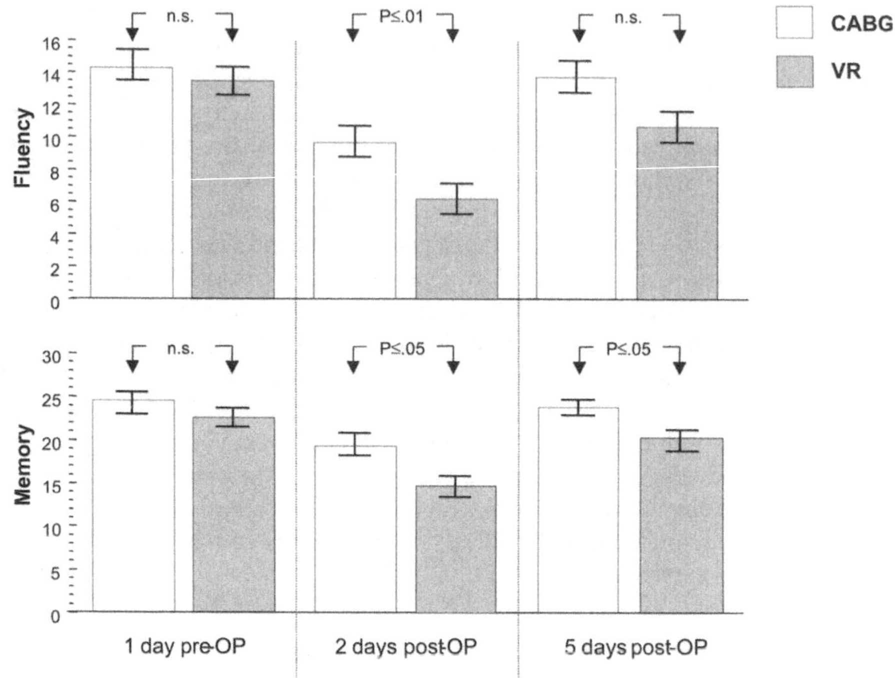

Fig. 4. A comparison of pre- and postoperative verbal fluency and memory disorders in coronary artery bypass grafting and valve replacement surgery (bars represent means ±SEM).

dergoing VR or CABG surgery. Again, both groups were exactly matched for age, sex, and the preoperative neuropsychological performance. The patients were assessed on the last or next to the last preoperative day, on the 2nd and 7th postoperative day and half of the patients were reexamined 6 months after surgery. Both patient groups did not differ with respect to known risk factors of postoperative neurobehavioral disorders (e.g., history of neurologic or psychiatric disorders or alcohol or drug abuse), and no patient showed an adverse neurologic outcome. A detailed analysis of the neuropsychological performance indicated that deficits were mainly observed in verbal memory and verbal fluency tasks. In contrast to bypass patients who showed no significant difference between preoperative and one week postoperative memory performance, patients undergoing valve replacement surgery continued to display a significant memory disorder one week after surgery. Six months later, however, we found no significant differences within or between groups.

Both, the data of the first and the second study indicate that patients undergoing valve replacement show more neuropsychological disorders and a slower recovery during the postacute stage after surgery. Verbal memory and verbal fluency were those neuropsychological domains affected most in both patient groups. This finding led to the hypothesis that a transient dysfunction of temporal lobe structures might be a functional correlate of an impaired neuropsychological performance after cardiac surgery under cardiopulmonary bypass conditions.

Hippocampal dysfunction as the functional correlate of postoperative neuropsychological disorders

Memory performance is highly dependent on the integrity of medial temporal lobe structures, and verbal fluency - mostly interpreted as a frontal lobe-associated function - was also shown impaired in patients with temporal lobe lesions. There is a huge number of studies on experimental ischemia in animals (3) or cell cultures (1) giving evidence that hippocampal neurons (Fig. 5) show a selective vulnerability to transient hypoxia.

This line of argument leads to the hypothesis that neuropsychological disorders after cardiac surgery could be predominantly attributed to temporal lobe dysfunction. Patients undergoing intracardiac operations seem to be especially vulnerable for neurobehavioral disorders due to a higher risk of transient ischemia (e.g., caused by cerebral microemboli). Microembolic signals are significantly more often detected in patients with valve replacement surgery compared to bypass grafting (16) and a recent study from Braekken and coworkers (2) demonstrated a significant association between postoperative neuropsychological deficits and the number of intraoperative microembolic signals only in VR patients. Another study from Jacobs and coworkers (6), however, was not able to replicate these findings. The authors reported no significant correlation between the number of high-intensity signals as-

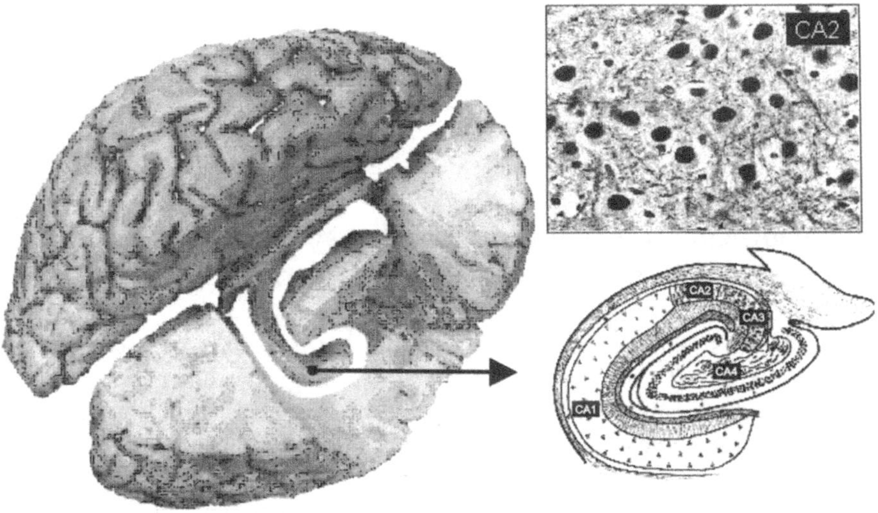

Fig. 5. The hippocampal formation: a brain structure with selective vulnerability to hypoxia.

sessed by transcranial ultra Doppler sonography and deficits in postoperative neuropsychological function or alterations in cerebral glucose metabolism. The study, however, consisted only of 2 patients who underwent VR surgery. Cerebral hypoxia – regardless of the cause – might play a major part in the etiopathogenesis of postoperative neurobehavioral alterations. This fact was also pointed out by Nollert and coworkers (11) who demonstrated by using near infrared spectroscopy that patients with neuropsychological deficits after cardiac surgery showed significantly reduced oxidized cytochrome a,a3 during operation.

Additional evidence for a higher risk of cerebral damage leading to neurobehavioral disorders in intracardiac operation came from a recent study of our research group. In this study (5) we aimed at a contrastive analysis of release patterns of neurobiochemical markers of brain damage after CABG and VR and their association with the postoperative neurobehavioral outcome. We analyzed neuron-specific enolase (NSE) and protein S-100B concentrations in serial venous blood samples taken preoperatively and 1, 6, 20 and 30 hours postoperatively in 18 patients with intracardiac operations (VR) and 18 patients undergoing isolated CABG surgery. Again, both groups were matched for age, sex, and preoperative cognitive performance. Both, VR and CABG patients, showed a significant increase of S-100B and NSE concentrations followed by a significant decrease during the next 30 hours. Whereas S-100B values did not differ significantly between patient groups, subjects undergoing VR surgery exhibited higher NSE values during the whole postoperative course (see Fig. 6). Furthermore, VR patients showed a higher decline in cognitive performance which was also detectable half a year after surgery. We found a significant correlation between the degree of individual postoperative decline of cognitive performance and S-100B area under curve values only in VR patients. These data gave additional evidence for the type of surgery representing a risk factor for postoperative neurobehavioral disorders. Furthermore, the data gave a first indication that the different vulnerability of neurobehavioral disorders might be mirrored in different postoperative release patterns of neurobiochemical markers of brain damage.

Neurobiochemical markers of brain damage and their association with postoperative neurobehavioral disorders

In recent years neurobiochemical markers of brain damage gained particular attention to identify patients with adverse neurological outcome after cardiac surgery. Due to commercial availability and non-invasive clinical applicability neuron-specific enolase (NSE) and protein S-100B are those markers of brain damage which have been studied most often in clinical and experimental settings. Neuron-specific enolase (NSE) is a dimeric isoenzyme of the glycolytic enzyme enolase predominantly found in the cytoplasm of neurons and cells

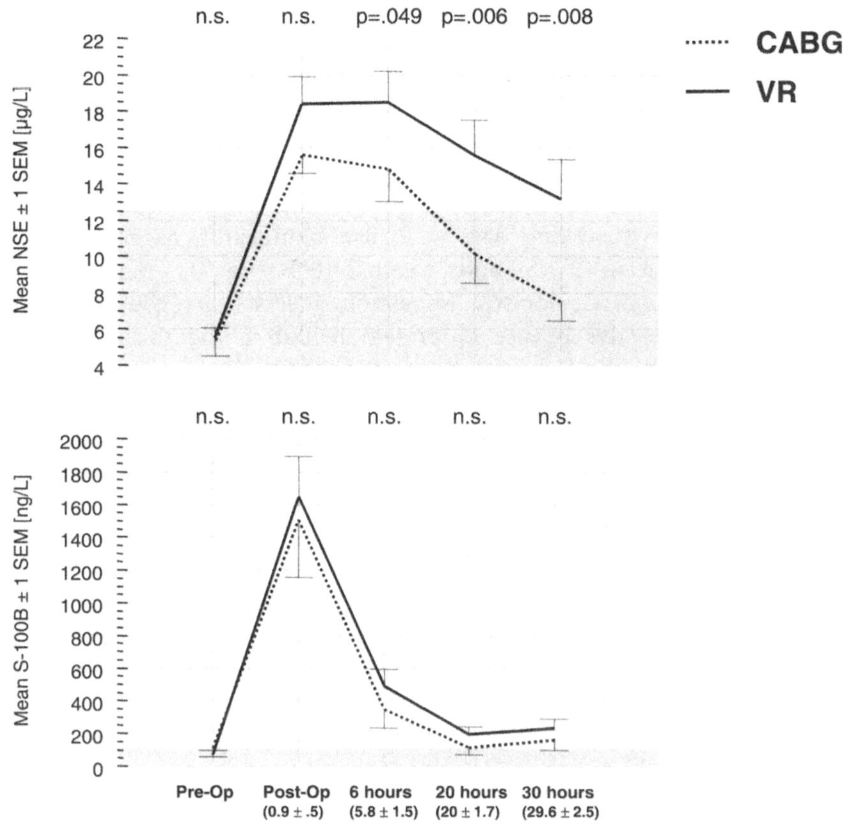

Fig. 6. Comparison of release patterns of neuron-specific enolase (NSE, top) and protein S-100B (bottom) in patients undergoing valve replacement and coronary artery bypass surgery (modified from (5)) matched by sex, age, and the preoperative cognitive performance. The marked area indicates the respective reference range of 95% of healthy control subjects.

with neuroendocrine differentiation (8). The enzyme is not secreted into the extracellular liquid by intact neurons but set free by cell destruction. Protein S-100B forms part of a large and diverse family of Ca^{2+}-binding proteins predominantly found in astrocytes and Schwann cells (13). The protein is secreted predominantly by astroglial cells and its release is considered to be associated with functional disturbance of membrane integrity and increased permeability of the blood-brain barrier.

In a broader study consisting of 66 patients undergoing elective cardiac surgery (53 patients with CABG and 13 patients with VR) we aimed at the analysis of the predictive value of NSE and protein S-100B for the short- and long-term neurobehavioral outcome. NSE and protein S-100B were sampled as described in the previous section and analyzed using monoclonal sandwich immunoluminometric assays (Sangtec®, Byk-Sangtec Diagnostica, Dietzenbach, Germany). All patients were examined pre- and postoperatively and half a year after surgery with detailed neuropsychiatric (DSM-III R, Brief Psychiatric and Delirium Rating Scale) and neuropsychological assessments (including orientation/global cognitive screening, memory functions, visuoperceptive/constructive functions, attentional performance, and executive functions). Patients who postoperatively exhibited a delirious state according to DSM-III R criteria presented significantly elevated postoperative serum concentrations of both NSE and protein S-100B. Neuropsychological deficits during the first 3 postoperative days were also significantly associated with elevated release patterns of NSE and protein S-100B (Fig. 7).

Using a multivariate logistic regression analysis, we could demonstrate that the postoperative release of protein S-100B is significantly associated with neuropsychological deficits two to three days after surgery. At this time,

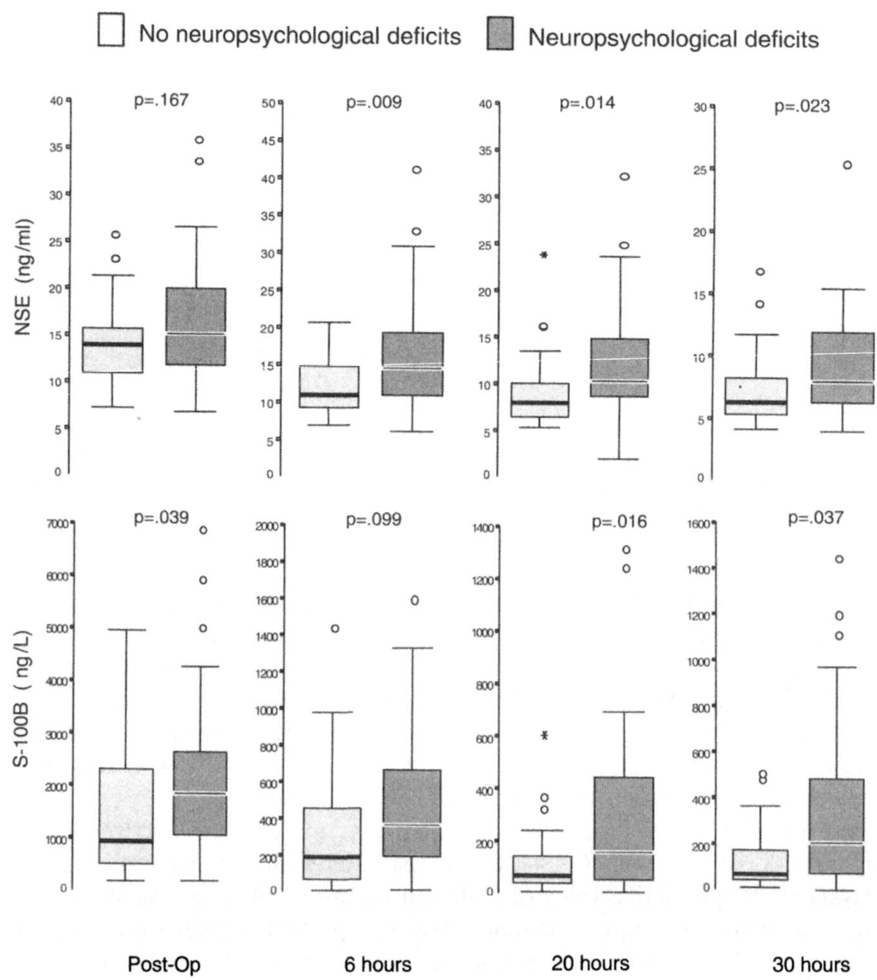

Fig. 7. Release patterns of neuron-specific enolase (NSE, top) and protein S-100B (bottom) in patients with and without neuropsychological deficits 3 days after cardiac surgery.

a low postoperative cardiac index, postoperative tachycardia, and low systolic blood pressure also contributed significantly to an adverse neuropsychological outcome. However, when analyzing the relation between the postoperative release of neurobiochemical markers and the long-term neuropsychological deficits, no significant association could be established.

Taken together, these findings clearly indicate that neurobiochemical markers of structural or functional brain damage can predict adverse postoperative neuropsychological outcome. But they also indicate that biochemical markers of brain damage may explain only part of the pathophysiological process underlying neurobehavioral alterations after cardiac surgery.

Summary

Heart surgery under cardiopulmonary bypass is one of the most frequently performed operations. Due to improvements in the cardiopulmonary bypass technique, cardiosurgical, anesthetic, and drug management, the relative number of patients with overt neurological complications has decreased. Neurobehavioral deficits after cardiac surgery, however, are reported to occur in a considerable high number of patients and pose a major impact on postoperative quality of live. As early as in the middle of the last decade Shaw and colleagues stated that "*there is abundant evidence that cardiac operations utilising cardiopulmonary bypass have become safer, when judged by the occurrence of fatal cerebral damage. We must now focus our attention on more subtle neurological complications, if further improvements are to be made*" (15). The data presented in this paper show that

- decreased neuropsychological function after cardiac surgery is found in about 50% of patients in the short-term and up to one fourth of patients in the long-time follow-up,
- patients undergoing valve replacement surgery are especially vulnerable to exhibit neurobehavioral disorders,
- type and degree of neuropsychological disorders are predominantly associated with cerebral structures highly vulnerable to hypoxia, and
- neurobiochemical markers of brain damage do predict part of the early neurobehavioral outcome after cardiac surgery and do mirror the underlying pathophysiology of neuropsychological dysfunction.

In order to further improve the long-term benefit of cardiac operations under cardiopulmonary bypass conditions, research focusing on the underlying cerebral pathophysiology of postoperative neurobehavioral disorders has to become a high priority topic in future research.

References

1. Bernaudin M, Nouvelot A, MacKenzie ET, Petit E (1998) Selective neuronal vulnerability and specific glial reactions in hippocampal and neocortical organotypic cultures submitted to ischemia. Experimental Neurology 150:30–39
2. Braekken SK, Reinvang I, Russel D, Brucher R, Svennevig JL (1998) Association between intraoperative cerebral microembolic signals and postoperative neuropsychological deficit: comparison between patients with cardiac valve replacement and patients with coronary artery bypass grafting. Journal of Neurology, Neurosurgery, and Psychiatry 65:573–576
3. Dijkhuizen RM, Knollema S, van der Worp HB, Horst GJ, Wildt DJ, Erkelbach van der R, Sprenkel JW, Tulleken KA, Nicolay K (1998) Dynamics of cerebral tissue injury and perfusion after temporary hypoxia-ischemia in the rat: evicence for region specific sensitivity and delayed damage. Stroke 29:695–704
4. Heller S, Kornfeld D (1986) Psychiatric aspects of cardiac surgery. Advances in Psychosomatic Medicine 15:124–139
5. Herrmann M, Ebert AD, Tober D, Huth C (1999) A contrastive analysis of release patterns of biochemical markers of brain damage after coronary artery bypass grafting and valve replacement and their association with the neurobehavioural outcome after cardiac surgery. Eur J Cardiothorac Surg (in press)
6. Jacobs A, Neveling M, Horst M, Ghaemi M , Kessler J, Eichstaedt H, Rudolf J, Model P, Bonner H, de Vivie ER, Heiss WD (1998) Alterations of neuropsychological function and cerebral glucose metabolism after cardiac surgery are not related only to intraoperative microembolic events. Stroke 29:660–667
7. Kuroda Y, Uchimoto R, Kaieda R, Shinkura R, Shinohara K, Miyamoto S (1993) Central nervous system complications after cardiac surgery: A comparison between coronary artery bypass grafting and valve surgery. Anesthesia and Analgesia 76:222–227
8. Marangos PJ (1987) Neuron specific enolase: A clinically useful marker of neurons and neuroendocrine cells. Annu Rev Neurosci 10:269–295
9. Murkin JM, Newman SP, Stump DA, Blumenthal JA (1995) Statement of consensus on assessment of neurobehavioral outcomes after cardiac surgery. Ann Thorac Surg 59:1289–1295
10. Newman S, Smith P, Treasure T, Joseph P, Ell P, Harrison M (1987) Acute neuropsychological consequences of coronary artery bypass surgery. Current Psychological Research Review 6:115–124
11. Nollert G, Möhnle P, Tassani-Prell P, Borasio GD, Schmoeckel M, Reichart B (1995) Postoperative neuropsychological dysfunction and cerebral oxygenation during cardiac surgery. Thoracic cardiovascular Surgeon 43:260–264
12. Roach GW, Kanchuger M, Mangano CM, Newman M, Nussmeier N, Wolman R, Aggarwal A, Marschall K, Graham SH, Ley C, Ozanne G, Mangano DT (1996) Adverse cerebral outcomes after coronary bypass surgery. The New England Journal of Medicine 335:1857–1863
13. Schäfer BW, Heizmann CW (1996) The S100 family of EF-hand calcium-binding proteins: Function and pathology. TIBS 21:134–140
14. Selnes OA, Goldsborough MA, Borowicz LM, McKhann GM (1999) Neurobehavioural sequelae of cardiopulmonary bypass. The Lancet 353:1601–1606
15. Shaw PJ, Bates D, Cartlidge NEF, French JM, Heaviside D, Julian DG, Shaw DA (1986) Early intellectual dysfunction following coronary bypass surgery. Quarterly Journal of Medicine 58:59–68
16. Thiel A, Zimmer M, Stertmann WA, Kaps M, Hempelmann G (1997) Microembolizations during heart surgery under extracorporeal circulation. Anaesthesiol Intensivmed Notfallmed Schmerzther 32:715–720
17. Walzer TA, Herrmann M (1998) Neuropsychologische und psychopathologische Veränderungen nach kardiochirurgischen Eingriffen. Fortschritte der Neurologie und Psychiatrie und ihrer Grenzgebiete 66:68–83

18. Walzer T, Herrmann M, Wallesch C-W (1997) Neuropsychological disorders after coronary bypass surgery. Journal of Neurology, Neurosurgery, and Psychiatry 62:644–648
19. Walzer TA, Wallesch CW, Starkstein SE, Herrmann M (1998) Neuropsychologische Defizite in der frühen postoperativen Phase nach kardiochirurgischen Eingriffen - Ein Vergleich zwischen Patienten mit Klappenersatz- und Bypass-Operationen. Zeitschrift für Neuropsychologie 9:123–132

Author's address:
Priv.-Doz. Dr. med. Dr. phil. Manfred Herrmann
Sektion Neuropsychologie mit neuropsychologischer
und verhaltensneurologischer Poliklinik
Otto-von-Guericke-Universität Magdeburg
Leipziger Str. 44
D-39120 Magdeburg, Germany

Clinical relevance of the systemic inflammatory reaction related to cardiac operations in children

M.-C. Seghaye[1], J. Vazquez-Jimenez[2], Ma Qing[1], B. Buding[3], J. Duchateau[4], B.J. Messmer[2], and G. von Bernuth[1]
[1] Department of Pediatric Cardiology, [2] Thoracic and Cardiovascular Surgery and [3] Anesthesiology, University Hospital Aachen, Germany and [4] Department of Immunology, Brugmann University Hospital, Brussels, Belgium

Introduction

Cardiac operations involving cardiopulmonary bypass (CPB) are related to a complex systemic inflammatory response which induces a variable degree of organ dysfunction. While CPB-related complications are relatively rare in adults undergoing elective cardiac surgery, postoperative organ dysfunction or multiple organ dysfunction syndrome remain important complications of pediatric cardiac surgery which are ascribed, at least in part, to the uncontrolled systemic inflammatory response (13).

The latter is mainly determined by the activation of the alternative pathway of the complement system due to the contact between blood and plastic surfaces (7, 8, 13). At the end of CPB, complement activation is enhanced by activation of the classical pathway by heparin-protamine complexes (12).

Activated complement proteins have a wide spectrum of biological effects. Particularly, they influence leukocyte function and are responsible for leukocyte mobilization, degranulation, and also for cytokine synthesis (31). Cytokine synthesis during CPB not only takes place in leukocytes but probably in virtually all nucleated cells: this has been shown for endothelial cells, hepatocytes, and cardiac myocytes (29, 30), activated by complement fragments and also by ischemia and reperfusion. This latter could probably be particularly important in young children undergoing cardiocirculatory arrest and in cyanotic patients undergoing corrective surgery with consecutive hyperoxygenation (3). Ischemia-reperfusion injury and pro-inflammatory cytokines are factors leading to the expression of adhesion molecules, enhancing in turn leukocyte-endothelial interactions (1, 2).

Mechanisms involved in the systemic inflammatory response in children undergoing cardiac surgery

Complement activation

In the setting of CPB, neonates and young children show significant C3- and C5-conversion (13, 18, 23, 24), indicating late phase activation of the complement system up to the terminal complex C5b-9 ("membrane attack complex"). Although neonates are known to have subnormal activity of the alternative pathway of complement, they behave similar when compared to older children (23). In our experience, significant complement activation is observed when rewarming the patient and ventilating the lungs with a maximal value at the end of the procedure (24). At this time point several simultaneous events take place: reinstitution of the myocardial perfusion, rewarming of the patient, and protamine administration. All these factors are well known to enhance complement activation.

Data from the literature are controversial with regard to the relationship between duration of CPB and magnitude of complement activation. Due to the number of factors involved in the complex reaction leading to complement activation, a strong relationship between the latter and the duration of the inflammatory stress is unlikely. The complement system shares several pathways and control mechanisms with other biological cascades involved in the pathophysiology of CPB, such as the plasma contact system, the coagulation system, and fibrinolysis (31), leading to the amplification of the inflammatory response.

Activated complement factors are potent activators of leukocytes and thus contribute to the propagation of the inflammatory stress by leading to leukocyte degranulation and cytokine synthesis (31).

Leukocyte degranulation

Leukocyte degranulation with release of proteases, such as elastase and myeloperoxidase or histamine, have been demonstrated in neonates and children undergoing cardiac surgery (22–24, 32). Central to the pathophysiology of CPB is also the release of oxygen-free radicals from neutrophils and endothelial cells. This is particularly important in patients with preoperative cyanosis who were shown to have reduced anti-oxidant activity when undergoing corrective surgery (3).

A strong relationship between degree of complement activation and leukocyte degranulation after CPB exists in children, which suggests a causative relationship between both phenomena (Fig. 1).

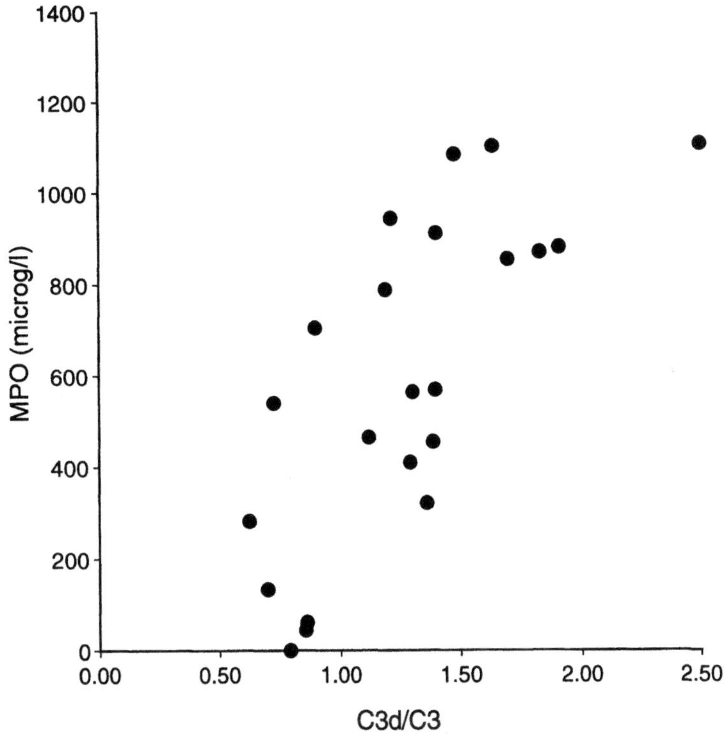

Fig. 1. Relationship between plasma concentrations of myeloperoxidase and C3d/C3 4 hours after CPB in 23 children. Spearman correlation coefficient 0.75, $p < 0.001$.

Cytokine synthesis

In the setting of pediatric CPB, activated leukocytes (particularly monocytes and granulocytes) express and release pro-inflammatory cytokines, which contribute to organ damage. Tumor necrosis factor-α, interleukin (IL)-6, and IL8 are usually considered cytokines with pro-inflammatory properties although IL6, which is the major regulator of the acute phase response, also has anti-inflammatory effects (9, 28). Neonates and children not only show a significant production of pro-inflammatory cytokines when submitted to cardiac surgery but also a natural anti-inflammatory response with production of IL10 (5, 11, 20). Usually, plasma concentrations of TNFα, IL6, and IL8 increase progressively and significantly during CPB, reaching maximal values at the end of the procedure, most likely due to the reasons exposed above. In contrast, liberation patterns of IL10 differ in the different reported pediatric series, either showing a peak at the end of CPB (27) or delayed, on the first postoperative day (20). This difference might be ascribed to perioperative management including, among others, pretreatment with corticosteroids (26) and degree of hypothermia during CPB (20).

While the exact mechanisms leading to cytokine synthesis during pediatric cardiac surgery are not fully understood, one can speculate that complement anaphylatoxins (31) and endotoxins released from the gut (10) trigger the pro-inflammatory cytokine production. Other mechanisms also have to be considered, such as hypoxia and reoxygenation, known to induce IL8 synthesis in vitro (19). As pro-inflammatory cytokines are inductors of IL10, it is likely that the natural anti-inflammatory response that follows the release of pro-inflammatory cytokines controls the latter, in an effort of the organism to maintain its homeostasis.

TNFα, IL1β, and IL8 are potent inductors of adhesion molecules expression, which in turn increase leukocyte-endothelial interactions, contributing to increased microvascular permeability and organ damage (6, 16, 17). Furthermore, they also exert their harmful effects by inducing the nitric oxide (NO) synthase and the production of non-physiological amounts of NO in the tissue.

Clinical implications of the systemic inflammatory reaction related to cardiac operations

Capillary leak syndrome

Capillary leak syndrome (CLS) which is characterized by the development of non-cardiogenic generalized edema including fluid accumulation in the third space with pleural effusion and ascites (21) is a frequent complication of pediatric cardiac surgery. Neonates are particularly at risk to develop this, due to their facilitated fluid movement across the capillary membrane leading to rapid fluid shift from the intravascular into the extravascular space in case of fluid overload. Picture shows important CLS in a neonate having undergone arterial switch operation for transposition of the great arteries (Fig. 2).

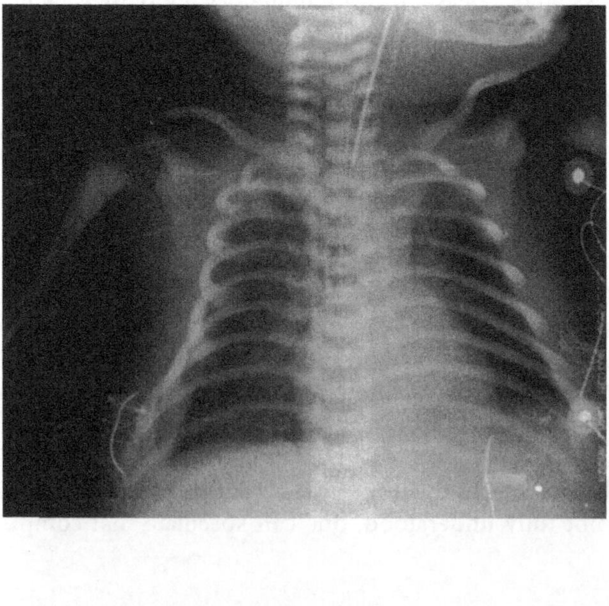

Fig. 2. Chest X-ray taken 48 hours after arterial switch operation in a neonate with transposition of the great arteries. This patient developed important CLS with generalized edema, pleural effusions, and ascites.

We investigated the role of the systemic inflammatory reaction on the development of CLS in a homogenous group of 24 neonates with transposition of the great arteries who underwent arterial switch operation (21). CLS developed in 13 of the 24 patients. Neonates with CLS had higher preoperative C5a plasma concentrations, higher preoperative leukocyte count, higher histamine, and TNFα release during CPB than those without CLS. Interestingly, patients with CLS showed significant higher capillary leakage with protein movement from the intravascular to the extra-vascular space as soon as 10 min after institution of CPB. These results suggested a close causal relationship between the magnitude of the systemic inflammatory response with release of inflammatory mediators increasing capillary permeability, and development of CLS in neonates. Furthermore, higher preoperative leukocyte count and C5a levels in patients developing CLS suggested an inflammatory state in those neonates, which could have been responsible for the priming of immune-competent cells during CPB and consecutive higher inflammatory response.

Loss of integrity of the endothelium is the ultrastructural substrate for tissue damage and finally for organ dysfunction related to CPB.

Multiple system organ failure

Multiple system organ failure (MSOF) is a syndrome which is thought to result from an uncontrolled systemic inflammatory reaction, as it occurs in the setting of sepsis, trauma, and major surgery (4). Cardiac operations with CPB are the major representatives of this latter category.

The absence of an accepted definition of MSOF in children experiencing MSOF after CPB led us to define it arbitrarily as the acute simultaneous occurrence in the first postoperative days with the failure of at least 2 vital organs in addition to cardiac insufficiency, thrombocytopenia, and high fever (25). In a prospective study designed to analyze the relationship between the systemic inflammatory reaction occurring during and after CPB and the development of postoperative MSOF, complement activation and leukocyte elastase release were measured before, during, and after CPB (24). Eight children out of the 29 investigated developed MSOF (27.5%). Patients with MSOF had significantly higher C3d/C3-ratios (as marker of C3-conversion) as early as during the rewarming phase than patients without MSOF. This higher complement activation in patients with MSOF persisted during the first postoperative week. Also leukocyte degranulation was significantly higher in children with MSOF as shown by the higher leukocyte elastase release in this group. All patients with MSOF had acute renal and hepatic failure in addition to cardiovascular insufficiency, thrombocytopenia, coagulation disorders, and high fever ($>39\,^{\circ}C$). Most of them also had transient arrhythmias (mostly junctional ectopic tachycardia), respiratory insufficiency, and neurological morbidity. Finally, in accordance with the high mortality related to MSOF commonly reported, 3 patients (37%) died postoperatively.

In this study, we were able to demonstrate the relationship between the degree of the systemic inflammatory response and the development of MSOF.

Transient postoperative arrhythmias

Transient postoperative arrhythmias such as junctional ectopic tachycardia, which classically occur after CPB and may spontaneously cease when the patient survives, are serious complications of surgery for congenital cardiac defects. They jeopardize the postoperative hemodynamic state mostly by the reduced ventricular filling period and by the loss of the atrio-ventricular sequence.

Histamine which is released during CPB from mast cells and circulating basophils (both targets for a large number of inflammatory mediators, i.e., complement anaphylatoxins and cytokines) has well-known arrhythmogenic properties (14). Histamine increases indeed spontaneous sinus rate, produces various degrees of atrioventricular block, and enhances the automaticity of ectopic pacemakers. A large number of in vitro and animal studies have demonstrated that histamine induces sinus tachycardia, junctional ectopic tachycardia, and ventricular tachycardia and that these effects are mediated through its H2 receptors (15).

In order to study the clinical relevance of histamine liberation during and after CPB with respect to the development of transient postoperative arrhythmias, we studied the course of histamine blood concentrations in 24 children, 8 of whom had transient postoperative arrhythmias (mainly junctional ectopic tachycardia) (22). In this study, patients with transient postoperaive arrhythmias had significantly higher histamine blood concentrations 4 hours after the operation than those without this complication. This observation suggests a causal relationship between the degree of histamine release during CPB and the occurrence of certain types of transient postoperative arrhythmias. Figure 3 shows an example of a junctional ectopic tachycardia in a

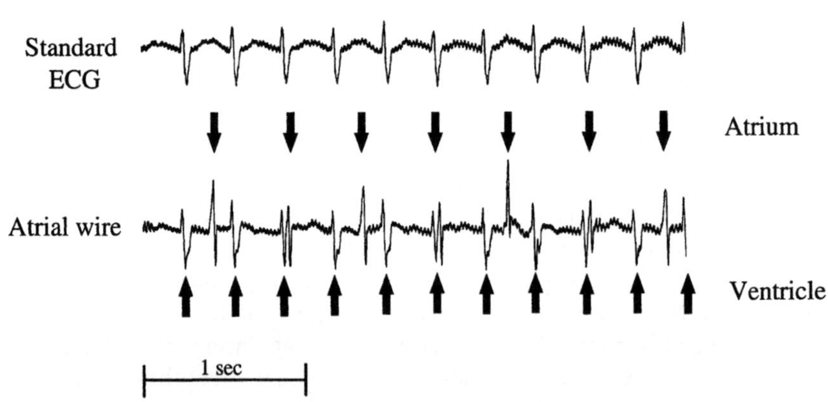

Fig. 3. Junctional ectopic tachycardia developing in a 1 month infant after CPB. In contrast to the standard ECG, the intracardial electrogram allows the diagnosis with narrow QRS complexes and an ventricular rate which is faster than the atrial one. The ventricular rate is about 220/min.

1 month old infant having undergone aorto-pulmonary shunt placement for pulmonary atresia.

Summary

Cardiac surgery involving CPB in children is related to a systemic inflammatory response comprising complement activation, leukocyte stimulation and degranulation, cytokine synthesis and increased leukocyte-endothelial interactions. Contact between blood and foreign surfaces during CPB and ischemia-reperfusion injury are probably the main inductors of this complex reaction of the organism primarily acting as a mechanism of homeostasis. Due to as yet nonclarified reasons, the systemic inflammatory reaction can become uncontrolled and then be the direct cause of specific morbidity. Complications such as capillary leak syndrome, multiple organ dysfunction syndrome, and certain types of transient postoperative arrhythmias are examples for this in neonates and young children.

Further work is necessary in order to reduce the specific CPB-induced postoperative morbidity, including the improvement of the extracorporeal circuits and pharmacological interventions which should modulate and control the systemic inflammatory response occurring during cardiac surgery.

References

1. Adams DH, Shaw S (1994) Leucocyte-endothelial interactions and regulation of leucocyte migration [see comments]. Lancet 343:831–836
2. Albelda SM, Smith CW, Ward PA (1994) Adhesion molecules and inflammatory injury. FASEB J 8:504–512
3. Allen BS, Rahman S, Ilbawi MN et al (1997) Detrimental effects of cardiopulmonary bypass in cyanotic infants: preventing the reoxygenation injury. Ann Thorac Surg 64:1381–1387
4. Anonymous (1992) American College of Chest Physicians/Society of Critical Care Medicine Consensus Conference: definitions for sepsis and organ failure and guidelines for the use of innovative therapies in sepsis [see comments]. Crit Care Med 20:864–874
5. Ashraf SS, Tian Y, Zacharrias S, Cowan D, Martin P, Watterson K (1997) Effects of cardiopulmonary bypass on neonatal and paediatric inflammatory profiles. Eur J Cardiothorac Surg 12:862–868
6. Brain SD (1994) Introduction: The Microcirculation. In: Brain SD (ed) Immunopharmacology of the Microcirculation. Academic Press, London San Diego New York Boston Sydney Tokyo Toronto, pp 1–7
7. Chenoweth DE, Cooper SW, Hugli TE, Stewart RW, Blackstone EH, Kirklin JW (1981) Complement activation during cardiopulmonary bypass: evidence for generation of C3a and C5a anaphylatoxins. N Engl J Med 304:497–503
8. Hammerschmidt DE, Stroncek DF, Bowers TK et al (1981) Complement activation and neutropenia occurring during cardiopulmonary bypass. J Thorac Cardiovasc Surg 81:370–377

9. Heinrich PC, Castell JV, Andus T (1990) Interleukin-6 and the acute phase response. Biochem J 265:621–636
10. Jansen NJ, van Oeveren W, Gu YJ, van Vliet MH, Eijsman L, Wildevuur CR (1992) Endotoxin release and tumor necrosis factor formation during cardiopulmonary bypass [see comments]. Ann Thorac Surg 54:744–747
11. Journois D, Israel-Biet D, Pouard P et al (1996) High-volume, zero-balanced hemofiltration to reduce delayed inflammatory response to cardiopulmonary bypass in children [see comments]. Anesthesiology 85:965–976
12. Kirklin JK, Chenoweth DE, Naftel DC et al (1986) Effects of protamine administration after cardiopulmonary bypass on complement, blood elements, and the hemodynamic state. Ann Thorac Surg 41:193–199
13. Kirklin JK, Westaby S, Blackstone EH, Kirklin JW, Chenoweth DE, Pacifico AD (1983) Complement and the damaging effects of cardiopulmonary bypass. J Thorac Cardiovasc Surg 86:845–857
14. Levi R, Owen DAA, Trzeciakowski J (1982) Actions of histamine on the heart and vasculature. In: Ganellin CR, Parsons ME (eds) Pharmacology of Histamine Receptors. Wright, PSG, Bristol London Boston, pp 236–297
15. Levi R, Zavecz JH (1979) Acceleration of idioventricular rhythms by histamine in guinea pig heart: mediation by H2 receptors. Circ Res 44:847–855
16. Liu JH, Djeu JY (1995) Role of cytokines in neutrophil functions. In: Aggarwal BB, Puri RK (eds) Human Cytokines: Their Role in Disease and Therapy. Blackwell Sciences, Cambridge Inc, MA, pp 71–86
17. Manogue K, van Deventer SJH, Cerami A (1991) Tumor Necrosis Factor Alpha or Cachectin. In: Thomson A (ed) The Cytokine Handbook. Academic Press Limited, London, pp 241–256
18. Meri S, Aronen M, Leijala M (1988) Complement activation during cardiopulmonary bypass in children. Complement 5:46–54
19. Metinko AP, Kunkel SL, Standiford TJ, Strieter RM (1992) Anoxia-hyperoxia induces monocyte-derived interleukin-8. J Clin Invest 90:791–798
20. Seghaye M, Duchateau J, Bruniaux J et al (1996) Interleukin-10 release related to cardiopulmonary bypass in infants undergoing cardiac operations. J Thorac Cardiovasc Surg 111:545–553
21. Seghaye MC, Grabitz RG, Duchateau J et al (1996) Inflammatory reaction and capillary leak syndrome related to cardiopulmonary bypass in neonates undergoing cardiac operations. J Thorac Cardiovasc Surg 112:687–697
22. Seghaye MC, Duchateau J, Grabitz RG et al (1996) Histamine liberation related to cardiopulmonary bypass in children: possible relation to transient postoperative arrhythmias. J Thorac Cardiovasc Surg 111:971–981
23. Seghaye MC, Duchateau J, Grabitz RG et al (1994) Complement, leukocytes, and leukocyte elastase in full-term neonates undergoing cardiac operation. J Thorac Cardiovasc Surg 108:29–36
24. Seghaye MC, Duchateau J, Grabitz RG et al (1993) Complement activation during cardiopulmonary bypass in infants and children. Relation to postoperative multiple system organ failure. J Thorac Cardiovasc Surg 106:978–987
25. Seghaye MC, Engelhardt W, Grabitz RG et al (1993) Multiple system organ failure after open heart surgery in infants and children. Thorac Cardiovasc Surg 41:49–53
26. Tabardel Y, Duchateau J, Schmartz D et al (1996) Corticosteroids increase blood interleukin-10 levels during cardiopulmonary bypass in men. Surgery 119:76–80
27. Tarnok A, Hambsch J, Schneider P (1998) Cardiopulmonary bypass-induced increase of serum interleukin-10 levels in children. J Thorac Cardiovasc Surg 115:475–477
28. Tilg H, Trehu E, Atkins MB, Dinarello CA, Mier JW (1994) Interleukin-6 (IL-6) as an anti-inflammatory cytokine: induction of circulating IL-1 receptor antagonist and soluble tumor necrosis factor receptor p55. Blood 83:113–118
29. Wan S, DeSmet JM, Barvais L, Goldstein M, Vincent JL, LeClerc JL (1996) Myocardium is a major source of proinflammatory cytokines in patients undergoing cardiopulmonary bypass. J Thorac Cardiovasc Surg 112:806–811

30. Wan S, LeClerc JL, Schmartz D et al (1997) Hepatic release of interleukin-10 during cardiopulmonary bypass in steroid-pretreated patients. Am Heart J 133:335–339
31. Weiler JM (1993) Introduction. In: Whaley K, Loos M, Weiler JM (eds) Complement in Health and Disease, 2nd ed. Kluwer Academic Publishers, Dordrecht, Boston, London pp 1–37
32. Withington DE, Elliot M, Man WK (1991) Histamine release during paediatric cardiopulmonary bypass. Agents Actions 33:200–202

Author's address:
PD Dr. Marie-Christine Seghaye
Medizinische Fakultät
Rheinisch-Westfälische Technische Hochschule
Pauwelsstraße 30
D-52057 Aachen, Germany
E-mail: mseghaye@post.klinikum.rwth-aachen.de

Procalcitonin (PCT) in cardiac surgery

M. Loebe, S. Lodziewski, F. Brunkhorst, C. Harke, and R. Hetzer
Department of Thoracic and Cardiovascular Surgery,
German Heart Centre, Berlin, Germany

Introduction

While markers of inflammatory response are very valuable for the detection and observation of infectious complications in general intensive care medicine (13), there are some distinct aspects of inflammation monitoring in patients undergoing open heart surgery procedures. Cardiac surgery is based on the use of extracorporeal circulatory circuits. The extended blood contact to foreign surfaces has a profound impact on the patient's milieu interne (5) and causes stimulation of the immune system (20, 32). In addition, most cardiac surgery institutions use hypothermia and low flow during extracorporeal circulation (ECC). All this may lead to profound alterations of inner organ perfusion as well as the patient's immuno-competence and immuno-response (37). Several authors were able to show complement activation, cytokine release, and other features of pro-inflammatory response during open heart surgery or immediately following the use of a heart lung machine (7, 8, 14, 20, 32). The use of extracorporeal circulation itself has been termed to be a cause of SIRS (systemic inflammatory response syndrome). Therefore, it may become extremely difficult to differentiate between infectious complications arising early after cardiac surgery and the general inflammatory response to the use of extracorporeal circulation. Since procalcitonin (PCT) has proved to be highly specific for bacterial and fungal infections (4, 10, 22), we investigated its course in patients undergoing cardiac operations. We measured PCT in patients in severe cardiogenic shock who had to be placed on biventricular support devices for life-saving reasons as well as a group of patients who received routine cardiac surgical procedures. We were interested to know whether this new marker of inflammation was unaltered by the use of extracorporeal circulatory circuits and whether profound cardiogenic shock with malperfusion of inner organs causes changes in the PCT level. Thereby, we hoped to determine the value of PCT in infection diagnosis and management early after open heart surgery as well as obtaining some further information about the pathophysiology that underlies the course of PCT levels.

Patients

Two cohorts of patients were studied. One group (VAD group) consisted of 39 patients aged 15 to 61 years (mean 40.8 years) who had to be implanted with a biventricular mechanical assist device Type Berlin Heart (Mediport GmbH, Berlin) (15) due to severe cardiac decompensation refractory to medical treatment. Device implantation was carried out using extracorporeal circulation and mild hypothermia. The VAD group was retrospectively subdivided according to the infectious status of the patient at the time before device implantation.

The second group (ECC group) consisted of 713 patients aged 16 to 87 years (mean 61.75 ± 11.9 years) undergoing routine cardiac operations. Again, mild hypothermia and the heart-lung machine were used during surgery in most cases.

Method

In the VAD group, the biventricular pneumatically driven pulsatile Berlin Heart assist device was used. This device consists of polyurethane-pumping chambers, mechanical heart valves, and silicon canullae connecting the extracorporeal VAD with the left and right atrium for blood drainage as well as with the ascending aorta and the pulmonary artery for returning the blood into the circulation. The use of the device, therefore, leads to extensive and continuous blood contact to foreign surfaces.

In the ECC group standard perfusion techniques were used with cardioplegic arrest (crystalloid cardioplegia) and mild hypothermia (28–32 °C). With

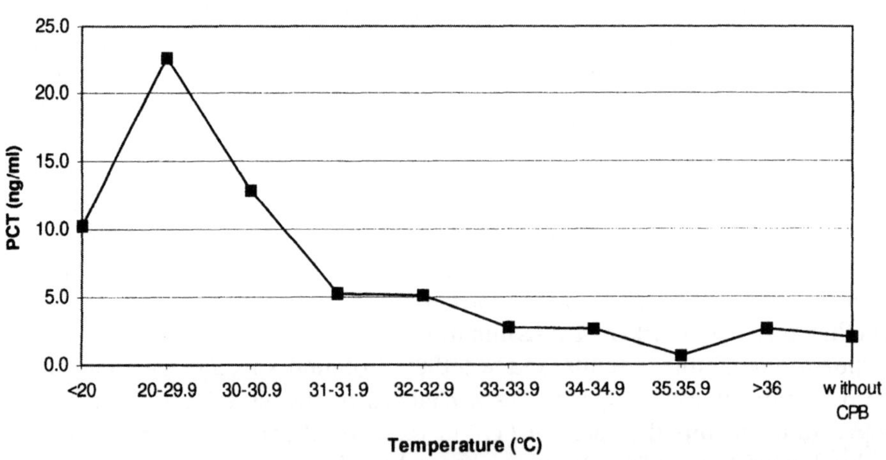

Fig. 1. PCT levels at the first day after surgery depending on deepest temperature reached during the procedure.

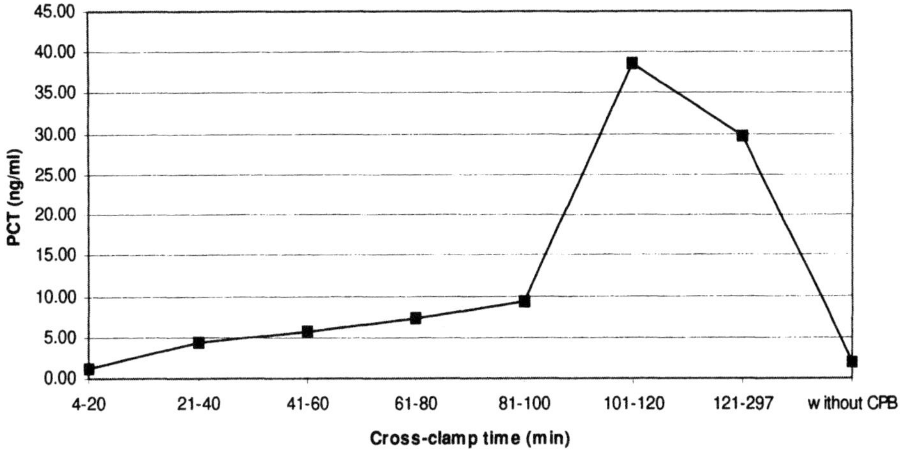

Fig. 2. PCT levels at the first day after surgery depending on the duration of aortic cross clamp time.

the exception of procedures involving the aorta, in general full flow perfusion was used.

Aortic cross-clamping time is the time the heart is arrested, while the perfusion time indicates the actual duration of ECC support. Patients were followed for 30 days after the open heart procedure.

Results

VAD group

Before device implantation, 17 patients had infections with positive blood cultures (subgroup A, n=9, and subgroup B, n=8). Thirteen had fever of unknown origin (subgroup D) and 9 patients were free from signs of infection (subgroup C). While 71% of the subgroup C reached heart transplantation (HTx) with a 100% survival after HTx, only 20% of the group A patients survived to transplantation. While all parameters of infection were significantly different between subgroups A and C, only PCT reached statistical significance when comparing patients in subgroup B (sepsis without shock) and in subgroup C (no infection). At the time of transplantation, none of the patients surviving the procedure showed elevated levels of PCT (0.1–0.3 ng/ml), while mean PCT level was 2.6 ng/ml in patients dying after transplantation.

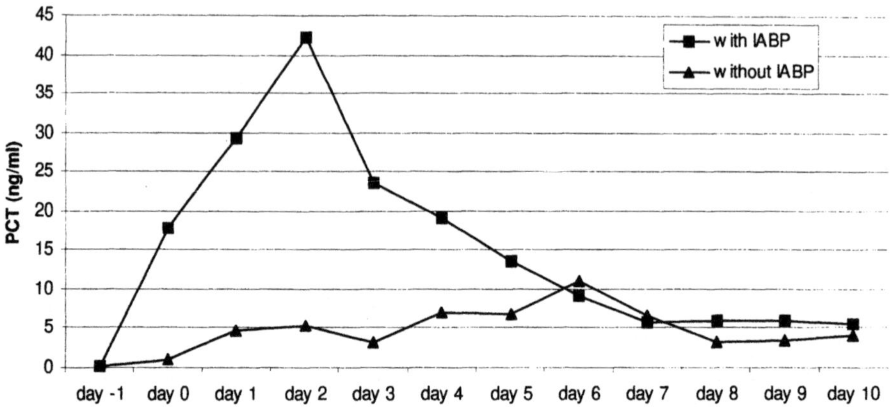

Fig. 3. Course of PCT in patients needing IABP support after surgery and those without hemodynamic compromitation.

ECC group

There were 512 coronary bypass surgery (CABG) patients of whom 94 (18%) patients underwent emergency operations for present or impending infarction. In 134 patients valve replacements and in 19 replacement of the thoracic aorta were carried out.

Mean aortic occlusion time was 48.47 min (max. 156 min) for CABG patients, 66.2 for valves (max. 297 min) and 83.11 min (max. 166 min) for thoracic aortic surgery patients. The mean perfusion time ranged from 104.5 min in CABG patients to 133.1 in valves and 164.2 min for aortic surgery.

Mean PCT levels before surgery were 0.165 ng/ml in CABG patients (max. 1.06 ng/ml), indicating that all CABG patients were free of infections before surgery. PCT levels rose to 2.42 ng/ml immediately after cardiac surgery reaching a peak at post-op day 5 with 10.48 ng/ml. However, 318 out of the 517 CABG patients (61%) had a PCT level below 1.0 ng/ml at day one after surgery while 100 (19%) had levels of more than 5 ng/ml.

The PCT level at day one after surgery was predictive of mortality: while 17 patients (17%) with PCT levels above 5 ng/ml died subsequently, only 3% of patients with PCT levels between 1 and 5 ng/ml at day one and 5 (1.6%) with normal PCT levels died.

In valve surgery patients, PCT before surgery was 0.52 ng/ml and rose to 1.614 ng/ml immediately after surgery reaching a peak with 12.30 ng/ml at the first day after operation. On the first day, 46 out of 134 patients (34%) had levels below 1.0 ng/ml and 50 patients (37%) had levels over 5.0 ng/ml.

Again, PCT levels at the first day after valve replacement predicted the further course of the patients. While in the group with PCT levels above 5 ng/ml 18% died; postoperative mortality was 5% for patients with moderately elevated PCT and 2% (n=1) in patients with normal PCT values.

Patients undergoing surgery of the intrathoracic aorta showed the most pronounced increase in PCT levels after open heart surgery. Mean PCT level before operation in this group was 0.411 ng/ml. Immediately after surgery with hypothermic circulatory arrest, it rose to 8.423 ng/ml. Finally PCT reached a peak at post op day 6 with 31.30 ng/ml. But again 35% of the patients in this group showed normal PCT levels at day one after surgery while 35% had levels of more than 5 ng/ml. While none of the patients with PCT under 1 died, one in the mildly elevated PCT group and 50% of patients with highly elevated PCT levels at the first day after operation died during the further postoperative course.

Discussion

The first part of our study demonstrated that PCT is able to identify concomitant bacterial infections in patients presenting with severe cardiogenic shock. Since identification of infections is extremely difficult and at the same time of outstanding importance in this group of moribund patients mostly presenting with fever, elevated WBC, and CRP due to cardiopulmonary congestion (3, 21, 38, 39), PCT had the unique property of predicting the patients further course. PCT was as well capable of identifying ongoing infections in patients on ventricular assist devices before transplantation, a feature which is important in defining the patients status of transplantability.

In the ECC group PCT levels before operation were within the normal range indicating that all patients were free of infections at this point in time. Nevertheless, an increase in mean PCT levels was observed immediately after use of the heart lung machine. However one third of the patients did not show any increase in PCT levels and this group had the most favorable prognosis after surgery. Interestingly this observation is independent of the type of surgery. It applies for elective CABG procedures as well as for valve replacements and extensive reconstructive surgery of the intrathoracic aorta. We believe that the increase of PCT in two thirds of our patients was due to diminished intestinal perfusion during the use of the heart lung machine. It seems that such an intestinal malperfusion caused endotoxin release by translocation as has previously been suggested as one of the possible reasons for PCT generation. Recently Kilger et al. (19) compared two small groups of patients undergoing coronary artery revascularization. One group was operated on using extracorporeal circulation while the second group underwent minimal invasive bypass surgery without the use of ECS. PCT levels were essentially normal in patients in whom ECS was not used. This again indicates that PCT release may well take place in the absence of bacterial or fungal infection. Our own data underline that nevertheless an elevated PCT level early after surgery indicates an increased risk for developing complications and an unfavorable further course. Only very few of our patients with increased PCT levels after surgery later on exhibited signs of infectious complications. The increased mortality in this group was mainly due to myocardial insufficiency.

These findings are very much in accordance with earlier observations on cytokine release during and after heart surgery (14, 20). It is well noted that the use of ECS causes profound stimulation of the proinflammatory response.

One may conclude from our findings that PCT is able to identify high risk patients early after cardiac surgery. It is worth considering specific therapeutical approaches such as broad spectrum antibiotics or immunomodulating medications in patients who show highly elevated PCT levels early after heart surgery and thereby improve the prognosis of this high risk population.

In the VAD group as well as in the ECC group the course of PCT levels was mostly independent from derangement originating from extensive blood contact with artificial surfaces and the use of extracorporeal circulation.

Several groups have previously demonstrated infections being a primary factor leading to morbidity and mortality in patients with assist devices as well as transplant recipients (1, 6, 9, 11, 18, 29, 34–36). While most groups would exclude patients with signs suggestive for infections from assist device implantation, we have tended to offer this treatment to all of those patients for whom no life saving alternative is in sight. Therefore, a large number of patients were included in this study who presented with fever and increased WBC. In our experience, PCT showed to be very helpful in diagnosing patients with ongoing systemic infections while on mechanical circulatory support. Transplantation was never considered as long as the patients showed signs of overt secondary organ dysfunction due to cardiogenic shock before device implantation (2, 12, 16, 18). This in combination with the shortage of donor organs led to increased periods of support time patients had to spend on the assist devices before being transplanted. But during these long waiting times many patients did develop local infections of the exit sites of the drivelines or canullas. In particular patients on left ventricular support devices who after being discharged home followed an active life faced this problem when their daily activities led to increased tension on the driveline and skin exit site (27). These patients are then in danger of infections ascending via the driveline into the pocket inside the abdominal wall where the ventricular assist device is located. Recurrent septic events originating from these infected pockets have been observed and pose a serious threat for the patients well-being (29, 30, 33). But possibilities of surgical intervention are limited and basically only complete removal of the infected device by heart transplantation can solve the problem (23, 28). Since patients then have to undergo immunosuppression, it is very dangerous to have uncontrolled infections present at the time of transplantation (24, 26). In our experience, PCT was highly elevated in the presence of systemic infection while localized infections at the skin exit site did not cause PCT elevation. Therefore, PCT can be used to determine if a given patient with drive line infection can be safely transplanted or if the antibiotic treatment needs to be intensified before the patient can be exposed to immunosuppression.

Conclusion

Procalcitonin was able to identify patients with ongoing bacterial infection while on mechanical assist devices. It was largely independent of the degree of cardiogenic shock before device implantation in patients in end stage heart failure. In patients undergoing conventional open heart surgery, one third did not show any PCT increase during or after use of extracorporeal circulation. However, one third of patients exhibited a pronounced increase of PCT after surgery. These patients tended to develop complications during their further postoperative course and had an increased mortality. Therefore, PCT was able to identify high risk patients early after open heart surgery. It may be very helpful in guiding the postoperative therapy in patients after open heart surgery and in choosing the optimal time point for transplantation in patients on mechanical assist devices.

References

1. American Heart Association (1995) Selection and treatment of candidates for heart transplantation. A statement for health professionals from the committee on heart failure and cardiac transplantation of the council on clinical cardiology. Circulation 92:3593–3612
2. Andresen B, Loebe M, Friedel N, Harke C, Ullmann H, Hetzer R (1997) Verlauf von Elastase, Komplementfaktor C3a und Endotoxin bei Patienten mit mechanischen extrakorporalen Kreislaufunterstützungssystemen Typ Berlin Heart. Z Herz, Thorax, Gefäßchir 11:100–107
3. Anker SD, Chua TP, Ponikowski P, Harrington D, Swan JW, Cox WJ, Poole-Wilson PA, Coats AJS (1997) Hormonal changes and catabolic/anabolic imbalance in chronic heart failure and their importance for cardiac cachexia. Circulation 96:526–534
4. Assicot M, Gendrel D, Carsin H, Raymond J, Guilbaud J, Bohoun C (1993) High serum procalcitonin concentration in patients with sepsis and infection. Lancet 341:515–518
5. Baier RE, Dutton RC (1969) Initial events in interactions of blood with foreign surfaces. J Biomed Mater Res 3:191–206
6. Bourge RC, Naftel DC, Costanzo-Nordin MR, Kirklin JK, Young JB, Kubo SH, Olivari MT, Kasper EK (1993) Pretransplantation risk factors for death after heart transplantation: a multiinstitutional study. J Heart Lung Transplant 12:549–562
7. Butler J, Chong GL, Baigrie RJ (1992) Cytokine responses to cardiopulmonary bypass with membrane and bubble oxygenator. Ann Thorac Surg 53:833–838
8. Chenoweth DE (1986) Anaphylatoxin formation in extracorporeal circuits. Complement 3:152–165
9. Costanzo MR (1996) Selection and treatment of candidates for heart transplantation. Seminars in Thoracic and Cardiovascular Surgery 8:113–125
10. DeWerra I, Jaccard C, Corradin SB, Chiolero R, Yersin B, Gallati H, Assicot M, Bohoun C, Baumgartner JD, Glauser MP, Heumann D (1997) Cytokines, nitrite/nitrate, soluble tumor necrosis factor receptors, and procalcitonin concentrations: comparisons in patients with septic shock, cardiogenic shock, and bacterial pneumonia. Crit Care Med 25:607–613
11. Frazier OH, Rose EA, MacManus Q, Burton NA, Tector A, Levin H, Kayne HL, Poirer VL, Dasse KA (1995) Improved mortality and rehabilitation of transplant candidates treated with a long-term implantable left ventricular assist system. Ann Surg 222:327–336

12. Friedel N, Viazis P, Schiessler A, Warnecke H, Hennig E, Tritin A, Bottner W, Hetzer R (1992) Recovery of end-organ failure during mechanical circulatory support. Europ J Cardio-thorac Surg 6:519–523
13. Gramm HJ, Hannemann L, Reinhart K, Lode H (1995) Sepsis: ein Begriff im Wandel. Möglichkeiten und Grenzen der Diagnose anhand klinischer Kriterien. Dtsch Med Wschr 120:498–502
14. Hammerschmidt DE, Stroncek DF, Bowers TK (1981) Complement activation and neutropenia during cardiopulmonary bypass. J Thorac Cardiovasc Surg 81:370–377
15. Hetzer R, Hennig E, Schiessler A, Friedel N, Warnecke H, Adt M (1992) Mechanical circulatory support and heart transplantation. J Heart Lung Transplant 11:175–181
16. Himmelreich G, Ullmann H, Riess H, Loebe M, Schiessler A, Hetzer R (1995) Pathophysiologic role of contact activation in bleeding followed by thrombembolic complications after implantation of ventricular assist device. ASAIO J 41:M790–M794
17. Hosenpud JD, Bennett LE, Keck BM, Fiol B, Novick RJ (1997) The registry of the International Society for Heart and Lung Transplantation: fourteenth official report-1997. J Heart Lung Transplant 16:691–712
18. Hummel M, Döcke WD, Friedel N, Baehr R v, Hetzer R, Volk HD (1994) Monitoring of cellular immune system in patients with biventricular assist devices awaiting cardiac transplantation. Clinical Transplantation 8:59–66
19. Kilger E, Pichler B, Goetz AE, Rank N, Welte M, Mörstedt K, Vetter HO, Gödje O, Schmitz C, Lamm P, Engerschalk E, Muehlbeyer D, Frey L (1998) Procalcitonin as a marker of systemic inflammation after conventional or minimally invasive coronary artery bypass grafting. Thorac Cardiovasc Surgeon 46:130–133
20. Kirklin JW, Westaby S, Blackstone EH (1983) Complement and the smaging effects of cardiopulmonary bypass. J Thorac Cardiovasc Surg 86:845–857
21. Kormos RL, Borovetz HS, Gasior T, Antaki JF, Armitage JM, Pistas JM, Hardesty RL, Griffith BP (1990) Experience with univentricular support in mortally ill cardiac transplant candidates. Ann Thorac Surg 49:261–272
22. Loebe M, Brunkhorst FM, Heinz U, Hetzer R (1996) Procalcitonin identifies bacterial sepsis in patients awaiting heart transplantation (Htx). Cardiovascular Surgery (Supple I):77 (Abstr)
23. Loebe M, Hennig E, Müller J, Spiegelsberger S, Weng Y, Hetzer R (1997) Long-term mechanical circulatory support as a bridge to transplantation, for recovery from cardiomyopathy, and for permanent replacement. Europ J Cardio-thorac Surg 11 Suppl:S18–24
24. Loebe M, Hetzer R, Schüler S, Hummel M, Friedel N, Weng Y, Schiessler A (1992) Herztransplantation – Indikation und Ergebnisse. Zentrbl Chir 117:681–688
25. Loebe M, Hummel M, Musci M, Sodian R, Grauhan O, Hetzer R (1995) Aktuelle Aspekte der Immunsuppression nach intrathorakalem Organersatz. Transplantationsmedizin 4:200–204
26. Loebe M, Schüler S, Spiegelsberger S, Matheis G, Warnecke H, Hetzer R (1990) Infektionen nach Herztransplantationen. Z Herz, Thorax, Gefäßchir 4:196–204
27. Loebe M, Weng Y, Müller J, Dandel M, Halfmann R, Spiegelsberger S, Hetzer R (1997) Successful mechanical circulatory support for more than two years with a left ventricular assist device in a patient with dilated cardiomyopathy. J Heart Lung Transplant 16:1176–1179
28. Massad MG, McCarthy PM, Smedira NG, Cook DJ, Ratliff NB, Goormastic M, Vargo RL, Navia J, Young JB, Stewart RW (1996) Does successful bridging with the implantable left ventricular device affect cardiac transplantation outcome? J Thorac Cardiovasc Surg 112:1275–1283
29. McCarthy PM, Portner PM, Tobler HG et al. (1991) Clinical experience with the Novacor ventricular assist system. J Thorac Cardiovasc Surg 102:578–587
30. Mehta SM, Aufiero TX, Pae WE Jr, Miller CA, Pierce WS (1995) Combined registry for the clinical use of mechanical ventricular assist pumps and the total artificial heart in conjunction with heart transplantation: sixth official report-1994. J Heart Lung Transplant 14:584–593

31. Meisner M, Tschaikowsky K, Schmidt J, Schüttler J (1996) Procalcitonin (PCT)-indications for a new diagnostic parameter of severe bacterial infection and sepsis in transplantation, immunosuppression and cardiac assist devices. Cardiovasc Engineering 1:67–76
32. Menache P, Haydar S, Peynet J (1994) One potential mechanism of vasodilatation after warm heart surgery: the temperature-dependent release of cytokines. J Thorac Cardiovasc Surg 107:293–299
33. Noon GP (1993) Clinical use of cardiac assist devices. In: Akutzu T, Koyanagi H (eds) Heart replacement: Artificial heart 4, Tokyo, Japan. Springer, pp 195–205
34. Pasic M, Loebe M, Hummel M, Grauhan O, Hofmeister J, Weng Y, Hetzer R (1996) Heart transplantation: a single-center experience. Ann Thorac Surg 62:1685–1690
35. Rose EA, Goldstein DJ (1996) Wearable long-term mechanical support for patients with end-stage heart disease: a tenable goal. Ann Thorac Surg 61:399–402
36. Rose EA, Levin HR, Frazier HO, Burton NA, Lefrak EA (1994) Artificial circulatory support with textured inner surfaces. Circulation 90:II87–91
37. Schirmer WJ, Schirmer JM, Naff GB, Fry DE (1988) Systemic complement activation produces hemodynamic changes characteristic of sepsis. Arch Surg 123:316–321
38. Smart FW, Naftel DC, Constanzo MR, Levine TB, Pelletier GB, Yancy CW, Hobbs RE, Kirklin JK, Bourge R (1996) Risk factors for early, cumulative and fatal infections after heart transplantation: a multiinstitutional study. J Heart Lung Transplant 15:329–341
39. Torre-Amione G, Kapadia S, Schort D, Young JB (1996) Evolving concepts regarding selection of patients for cardiac transplantation – assessing risks and benefits. Chest 109:223–232

Author's address:
Dr. M. Matthias Loebe
Klinik für Thorax- und Kardiovaskularchirurgie
Deutsches Herzzentrum Berlin
Augustenburger Platz 1
D-13353 Berlin, Germany

GPSR Compliance

The European Union's (EU) General Product Safety Regulation (GPSR) is a set of rules that requires consumer products to be safe and our obligations to ensure this.

If you have any concerns about our products, you can contact us on ProductSafety@springernature.com

In case Publisher is established outside the EU, the EU authorized representative is:

Springer Nature Customer Service Center GmbH
Europaplatz 3
69115 Heidelberg, Germany

Batch number: 10577876

Printed by Printforce, the Netherlands